The Eye in Primary (
A Symptom-based Appro

To Pippa, Nairn and Rory

Commissioning editor : Melanie Tait
Development editor : Zoë A. Youd
Production Controller : Chris Jarvis
Desk editor : Claire Hutchins
Cover designer : Fred Rose

The Eye in Primary Care:

A Symptom-based Approach

Hunter Maclean
FRCS, FRCOphth

Consultant Ophthalmologist
Queen Alexandra Hospital
Portsmouth, UK

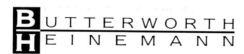 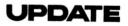

OXFORD   AUCKLAND   BOSTON   JOHANNESBURG   MELBOURNE   NEW DELHI

Butterworth-Heinemann
Linacre House, Jordan Hill, Oxford OX2 8DP
225 Wildwood Avenue, Woburn, MA 01801-2041
A division of Reed Educational and Professional Publishing Ltd

⟨R⟩ A member of the Reed Elsevier plc group

First published 2002

© Reed Educational and Professional Publishing Ltd 2002

British Library Cataloguing in Publication Data
A catalogue record for this book is available from the British Library

Library of Congress Cataloguing in Publication Data
A catalogue record for this book is available from the Library of Congress

ISBN 0 7506 5288 8

For information on all Butterworth-Heinemann publications
visit our website at www.bh.com

Composition by Scribe Design, Gillingham, Kent, UK
Printed and bound in Italy

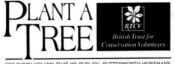

FOR EVERY VOLUME THAT WE PUBLISH, BUTTERWORTH-HEINEMANN
WILL PAY FOR BTCV TO PLANT AND CARE FOR A TREE.

Contents

Preface

Patients see their doctor with symptoms, and not with anatomical descriptions of where their complaints originate. This is the basic axiom of this book, and as a result I have attempted to cover the majority of symptoms that patients may complain of. Each chapter is structured to help the primary care doctor arrive at the diagnosis or possible diagnoses for a particular symptom, and in particular to flag certain diseases that may be rare but have important consequences if there is delay in the diagnosis.

Inevitably the introductory chapters deal with the dry subject of anatomy and how to examine the eye – skip this bit if you already feel confident in this area, and use it to dip into occasionally for reference purposes.

Referral guidelines are included for certain common conditions, and there is a section on the optician's letter, which is a common pathway for referral into primary care.

The book has two further purposes. First, it gives information especially about eye operations in order to arm the primary care physician with the knowledge to answer questions posed by anxious patients. Second, information is given, including a section on miscellaneous words, drugs and rarities, to furnish the reader with a means of interpreting letters from the ophthalmologist!

Hunter Maclean

Acknowledgements

Acknowledgement is due to:

Adam Booth, who took time to review the manuscript and point out any errors and inconsistencies.

Diane Forster, Pam Johnson and Emma Stacey, who were of great help in compiling the chapters on childhood eye conditions.

My wife, Pippa, for spending many hours reviewing and correcting the manuscript and proofs.

Hector Chawla (*Ophthalmology: A Symptom-based Approach*, Butterworth-Heinemann, 1999), Jack Kanski (*Clinical Ophthalmology*, Butterworth-Heinemann, 1999), R.D. Finlay and P. A. Payne (*The Eye in General Practice*, Butterworth-Heinemann, 1997) from whose books many of the illustrations were taken or adapted. Also Terry R. Tarrant whose illustrations are included from *Clinical Ophthalmology*.

Design of the eye

THE STRUCTURE OF THE EYE

The structure of the eye is analogous to that of a camera (Figure 1.1). The components required are:

● A strong outer box	The sclera
● A black internal lining to prevent internal reflections	The uveal tract
● A variable light aperture	The pupil reflex
● A lens	The cornea
● An adjustable focus	The crystalline lens
● Photographic film	The retina

Figure 1.1 Cross-section of an eye. The solid black area indicates the uveal tract.

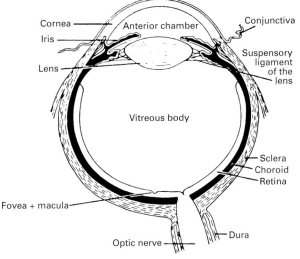

The sclera

The sclera (from the Greek *skleros*: hard) is a spherical, white, tough fibrous casing that surrounds the contents of the eye. It has two defects in its surface, one to allow passage of the optic nerve into the eye and the second to accommodate the cornea.

Associated disease:
- Inflammation
    Scleritis
    Episcleritis

The uveal tract

The uveal tract (from the Latin *uva*: grape) consists of the pigmented parts of the eye, with its name deriving from its grape-like appearance after the sclera has been removed. It is made up of melanocytes, and is split into three areas:

- The choroid – uveal tissue under the retina
- The ciliary body
    Pars plana – an intermediate joining piece
    Pars plicata – origin of the suspensory zonules of the lens
- The iris.

The choroid is very vascular, and nourishes the overlying retina. The choroid and retina are shaped like a brandy glass (see Figure 1.1), where the rim of the glass marks the end of the retina and choroid and the beginning of the pars plana. As the name suggests, the pars plana is plain and has no important structures within it. This is of great advantage to eye surgeons as it gives them an area where they can safely gain access to the posterior part of the eye – for example, to perform a vitrectomy (Figure 1.2). After about 4 mm the pars

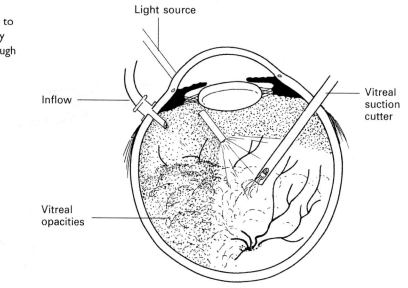

Figure 1.2 Vitrectomy for vitreous haemorrhage. Access to the vitreous cavity is gained by inserting the instruments through the pars plana.

Light source

Inflow

Vitreal suction cutter

Vitreal opacities

plana runs into the pars plicata, which (as its name suggests) is thrown into plicated folds similar to the villi of the intestine. These plicated folds are the origin of the zonules that suspend the lens in the centre of the eye, while the covering epithelium of the pars plicata produces aqueous. The final part of the uveal tract is the iris, which can constrict (a parasympathetic response and therefore stimulated by acetylcholine) and dilate (a sympathetic response and therefore stimulated by adrenaline) and so control the amount of light entering the eye via the pupillary reflexes.

Associated disease:
● Inflammation
  Choroid – choroiditis (posterior uveitis)
  Ciliary body – cyclitis (intermediate uveitis)
  Iris – iritis (anterior uveitis)
● Tumours
  Melanoma

Figure 1.3 The direct and consensual pupil response. Light is transmitted to the occipital cortex via the optic nerve, chiasm, optic tract and optic radiation. A connection to the midbrain stimulates parasympathetic nerve fibres, which hitchhike with the third nerve and cause pupillary constriction of both eyes.

The pupil reflex

To reduce the amount of light entering the eye, the iris constricts if illuminated ('the direct response'). This occurs by virtue of a synapse in the brain that connects the optic tract with the midbrain (Figure 1.3). Once stimulated, the midbrain sends a signal to the irises of both eyes to constrict even if only one eye was illuminated ('the consensual reflex'). The

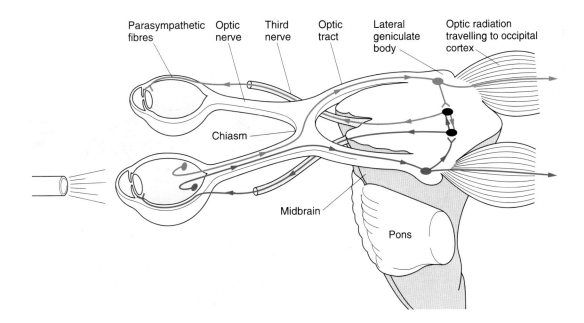

Parasympathetic fibres Optic nerve Third nerve Optic tract Lateral geniculate body Optic radiation travelling to occipital cortex

Chiasm

Midbrain

Pons

pupil of a normal eye will briskly constrict if illuminated; if it does not, it is abnormal (see Examination technique, below).

The cornea

The cornea is a truly specialized structure. It is totally transparent and contains no blood vessels, deriving its oxygen supply from the atmosphere instead. In health it is crystal clear and made up of three layers:

- Epithelium – when removed, for example during an abrasion, this has the ability to regenerate
- Stroma – if this is injured, healing occurs by scarring
- Endothelium – this consists of a single layer of cells, which are responsible for the deturgescence ('dehydration') of the cornea. Once destroyed, they do not regenerate.

Corneal clarity depends upon corneal dehydration. If sufficient endothelial cells are damaged or destroyed, corneal hydration occurs with loss of corneal clarity. Substituting a donor cornea with a healthy population of endothelial cells (a corneal transplant) is the only way of rectifying this situation.

The cornea is also the most powerful refracting surface (lens) in the eye. This is because light rays refract (bend) most when travelling from air to a medium with a higher refractive index, such as the cornea.

Associated disease:
- Loss of epithelium
    Corneal abrasion
- Infection/inflammation ('keratitis')
    Bacterial ulceration
    Viral ulceration – e.g. herpetic dendritic ulcer
- Damage or loss of endothelial cells
    Corneal oedema
- Corneal dystrophy
    Keratoconus.

The crystalline lens

The crystalline lens is suspended in the centre of the eye by a 360° network of zonules in a fashion analogous to a circular trampoline. The zonules are attached to the plicated surface of the ciliary body and the tension within them is influenced by the tone of the ciliary muscle, which is buried within the ciliary body. The ciliary muscle, shaped similarly

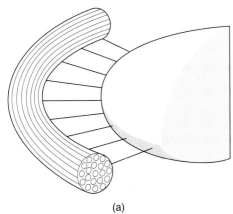

(a)

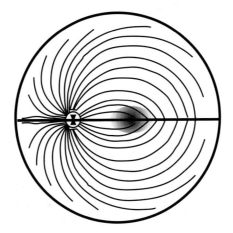

(b)

Figure 1.4 Accommodation. (a) With the ciliary muscle at rest, the zonules are taut. (b) Contraction of the ciliary muscle relaxes zonular tension, and the inherent elasticity of the lens causes it to increase in size and refractive power.

to a ring doughnut, is responsible for altering the shape of the lens and therefore its power via the tractional pull of the zonules. This process allows the eye to have a variable focus, which is needed to achieve both distance and near vision. Increasing the power of the lens to allow for near vision is known as accommodation (Figure 1.4). With age the lens becomes less distensible and so progressively less power is generated by accommodation, and thus the ability to focus on objects up close is gradually lost ('presbyopia'). Reading glasses are typically required at around 45 years of age.

Associated disease:
● Clouding of the lens
    Cataract.

The retina

The retina is made up of millions of photoreceptors (rods and cones), which are most concentrated in the macular area. The

Figure 1.5 Arrangement of retinal nerve fibres. The nerve fibres respect the horizontal midline.

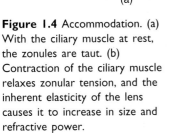

Figure 1.6 Diagram of the four major vascular arcades. The shaded area represents the macula.

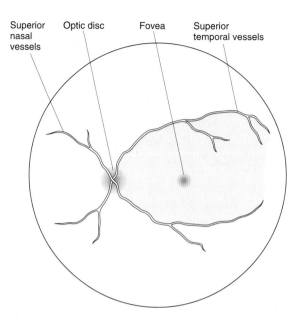

photoreceptors synapse with nerve fibres that collect at the optic nerve and travel to the visual centre in the occipital lobe of the brain. There is an overall pattern to the distribution of nerve fibres within the eye (Figure 1.5). The blood vessels also follow a consistent pattern. After the optic disc, the central retinal artery and vein split into four vascular arcades (Figure 1.6). The macular area is defined as the area bounded by the temporal artery and vein complex, and roughly conforms to a 'C' shape. The fovea is at the centre of the macula and is the point of greatest visual acuity.

Associated disease:
- Tearing
    - Retinal detachment
- Loss of function
    - Artery occlusion
    - Vein occlusion
    - Neuritis
- Ischaemia with new vessel formation
    - Vein occlusion
    - Diabetes
- Tumour
    - Retinoblastoma.

The vitreous

The vitreous (from the Latin *vitrum*: glass) fills up the posterior cavity behind the crystalline lens. It has the consistency of raw egg white, and there are no visual consequences if it is removed. With age it liquefies and collapses on itself, often causing symptoms of floaters.

Associated disease:
- Inflammatory cells in the vitreous
  Vitritis
- Collapse of the vitreous
  Posterior vitreous detachment.

The aqueous

The aqueous (from the Latin *aqua*: water) is a nutrient solution that bathes the anterior chamber of the eye, taking on the role normally performed by blood. After production by the ciliary epithelium it circulates through the pupil into the anterior chamber, and drains via the trabecular meshwork into the canal of Schlemm and onwards into the venous circulation (Figure 1.7).

Figure 1.7 Circulation of aqueous. The trabecular meshwork is a circular drain located in the angle of the anterior chamber at the junction of the iris root and cornea.

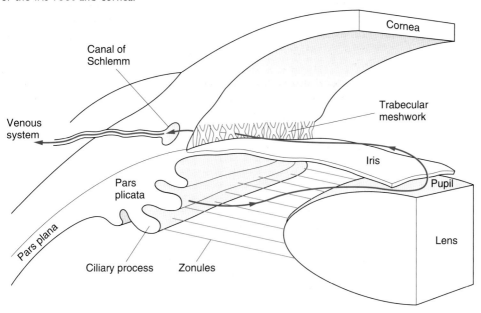

Associated disease:
- Blockage/obstruction of the meshwork
  Glaucoma.

EYE PROTECTION

The delicate structures of the eye are protected by:

- The bony orbit
- The eyelids and blink reflex
- Corneal sensation
- Reflex watering.

The bony orbit acts as armour plating, but the eye is still vulnerable to a straight-on attack by any object smaller than the orbital rim – for example, a squash ball. Corneal sensation (fifth nerve), which can trigger the blink reflex as well as reflex watering, provides further protective mechanisms.

The eyelids

The eyelids are moveable curtains composed of skin on the outside and conjunctiva on the inside. This allows them to glide over the corneal surface, gently washing its surface with tears and maintaining its optical clarity (Figure 1.8). The eyelids are kept in position by medial and lateral canthal tendons, which are attached to the bones of the orbit. Each lid contains dense formations of connective tissue called the tarsal plate, which also houses the meibomium glands. These glands secrete oil to stabilize the tear film, and have their

Figure 1.8 Cross-section of the eye within the orbit. Note that during eye closure only the top lid moves.

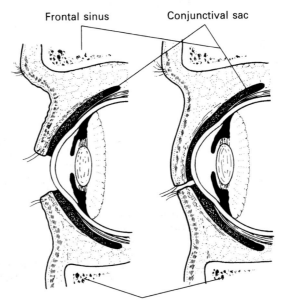

Frontal sinus   Conjunctival sac

Maxillary sinus

orifices on the lid margin. Tears collect on the bottom lid and drain out via the puncti to the nasolacrimal duct, which exits into the nose. This is why it is possible to taste tears or any medication that is placed into the eye.

Associated disease:
- Laxity of the canthal tendons
    Ectropion/entropion
- Blockage of the meibomium orifices
    Meibomium cyst/chalazion
- Blockage of the nasolacrimal duct
    Chronic watering eye.

THE NORMAL EXTERNAL EYE

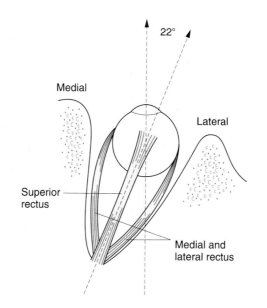

The upper eyelid forms an arc that obscures approximately 1 mm of iris (Figure 1.9). Any scleral show between the top of the iris and the upper lid is indicative of lid retraction. The position of the lower lid is more variable, but it usually obscures the inferior edge of the iris. Scleral show is not necessarily pathological.

HOW THE EYE MOVES

Figure 1.9 Normal external eye.

There are six extraocular muscles, four recti and two obliques, which move the eye. There is often confusion over the actions of these muscles on the eye, and this arises because the eye

Figure 1.10 Action of the superior rectus muscle.

22°

Medial

Lateral

Superior rectus

Medial and lateral rectus

and its muscles are frequently viewed out of context. It would appear self-evident that the superior rectus ought to move the eye directly upward – that is, until you put the eye in its normal setting. The key difference is that the orbits are angulated such that the superior rectus does not travel straight back from the eye but rather at an angle of approximately 22° (Figure 1.10). The result is that the action of the superior rectus moves the eye up and out. The inferior rectus, for the same reason, moves the eye down and out, while the medial and lateral recti move the eye as might intuitively be expected. The superior oblique muscle is the only muscle innervated by the fourth nerve, and its action is complicated by a pulley system (trochlear, the alternative name for the fourth nerve, means 'pulley'). The pulley alters the line of pull of the muscle such that when the eye is already looking toward the nose the action of the superior oblique is to pull the eye downwards (Figure 1.11). The inferior oblique has the opposite effect and moves the eye up and inwards (Figure 1.12). Coordination of eye movements so that each eye works in tandem with its partner occurs in the brainstem.

Associated disease:
● Muscular problems
    Thyroid eye disease
    Myositis
    Blow-out fracture

Figure 1.11 Action of the superior oblique muscle. When the eye looks toward the nose (b) activation of the muscle pulls the eye downward.

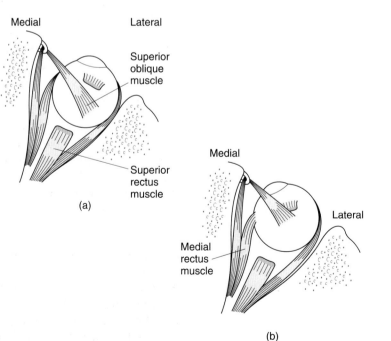

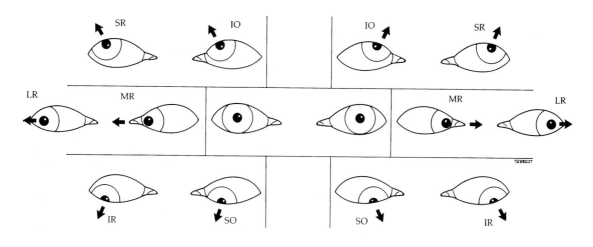

Figure 1.12 Action of all the extraocular muscles. Reproduced with permission from *Clinical Ophthalmology* by J. Kanski, 1999.

- Peripheral nerve dysfunction
    Cranial nerve palsies
- Central nervous system dysfunction
    Nystagmus
    Gaze palsies.

CENTRAL VISUAL ACUITY AND THE VISUAL FIELD

While the eye is analogous to a camera in structure, its function is slightly different. The camera takes a single picture with each point of the picture portrayed in equal detail. This is not so for the eye, where vision is continuous with only the central area portrayed in any detail. Each part of the retina has a particular sensitivity (to light) or visual acuity, and this is related to the density of photoreceptors in that area. These sensitivities can be plotted three-dimensionally, joining areas of equal sensitivity with a line ('isopter'), and the result is much like an Ordnance Survey map of a hill (Figure 1.13). The highest point and area of greatest sensitivity or visual acuity is the fovea, which is surrounded by a small area of lesser sensitivity, the macula. It is interesting to note how rapidly the sensitivity drops off with increasing distance from the fovea. The sensitivity in the periphery is in fact very primitive. This lack of sensitivity is easily demonstrated as follows:

- Take this book and once you have read these instructions close it.
- With your left eye closed, look straight ahead with your right eye.
- Now hold up the title page in your right hand, at arm's length and directly in front of you.

Figure 1.13 'Hill of vision'. Reproduced with permission from *Clinical Ophthalmology* by J. Kanski, 1999.

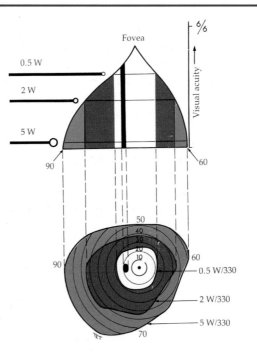

- Keeping your gaze fixed straight ahead and your arm outstretched, move the book in a slow arc toward the peripheral vision on the right-hand side.
- Notice how rapidly the detail on the book cover becomes completely indecipherable. By the time it reaches the periphery of the field it is no more than a shape.

There is a total blank spot in the graph 15° from the fovea, and this reflects the blind spot in the visual field. This exists because there are no photoreceptors on the optic disc. The blind spot is also easily demonstrated:

- Position yourself in front of a blank wall and close your left eye.
- Fix your right eye on a point of interest such as a dirty mark or the corner of a picture frame.
- With your right arm outstretched and your right hand in the 'thumbs up' position, line up your thumbnail with your chosen object of interest.
- Now, while keeping your right eye fixed on the point of interest, slowly move your right thumb to the right-hand side in the horizontal plane. After about 20 cm of travel, you will notice that the tip of your thumb has disappeared into the blind spot.
- If you now move your thumb in all directions until it reappears in your vision, you can map out the size of the blind spot.

Perhaps the most surprising thing is the size of the blind spot, which we do not appreciate on a day-to-day basis. This experiment gives you some insight as to why patients suffering from conditions such as glaucoma generally do not appreciate field defects until they are very large or impinge upon the central visual field.

THE VISUAL PATHWAY

With both eyes open, the visual field is split down the centre into the right- and left-hand sides (Figure 1.14). All the information from one side, which is contributed to by both eyes, is relayed to the contralateral occipital cortex. To achieve this,

Figure 1.14 The visual pathway.

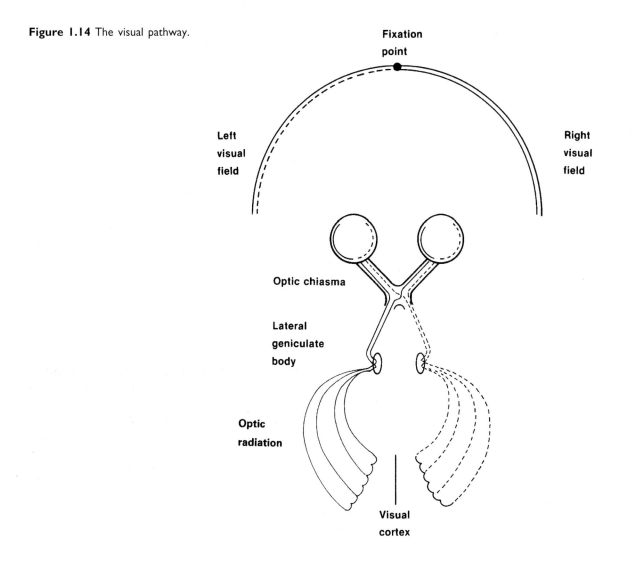

Fixation
point

Left
visual
field

Right
visual
field

Optic chiasma

Lateral
geniculate
body

Optic
radiation

Visual
cortex

50 per cent of the nerve fibres from each eye cross over to the other hemisphere at the chiasm. It is due to this arrangement that vascular accidents involving one occipital lobe result in loss of half of the visual field ('homonymous hemianopia') in both eyes.

Examination technique

Most doctors associate examination of the eyes with the ophthalmoscope, and a vague feeling of dread ensues. In fact, the eye can be successfully examined with a mixture of plain observation and some simple clinical tests, some of which involve the ophthalmoscope. However, if the ophthalmoscope is needed, the combination of a well-charged instrument and a dilated pupil makes a difficult manoeuvre achievable.

EQUIPMENT

The following equipment is required:

- A means of testing the visual acuity – ideally an illuminated Snellen chart placed 6 m from the patient.
- A light source – a pen torch, ophthalmoscope or auroscope will do.
- A magnifier – an ordinary magnifying glass or a standard auroscope without the speculum is useful (Figure 2.1).
- Fluorescein-impregnated paper strips (Fluorets®) – moistened with tears from the lower conjunctival sac, the dye will stain any defects of the corneal epithelium. This will

Figure 2.1 Examining the eye with a ×5 magnifying glass.

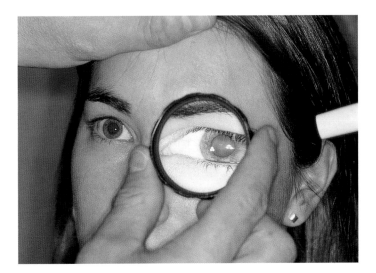

be even more obvious due to green fluorescence if a blue filter covers the light source.

- Dilating drops – tropicamide (Mydriacyl®) 1% is available in single-use containers as minims®/tropicamide. Do not use the fear of inducing acute glaucoma as an excuse for not dilating the pupil; few ophthalmologists do. The trick is to connect the two events if the patient complains of a sore red eye the next day, and refer immediately.
- Cotton buds – these are magnificent for removing corneal foreign bodies and everting eyelids and, if times are slow, relief from itchy ears.
- Anaesthetic drops – amethocaine drops, again available as single-dose minims, are useful to alleviate pain and blepharospasm and so allow examination. They should not be used as an ongoing treatment for pain, as they prevent healing.
- An ophthalmoscope – this is useful as a light source and for examining the red reflex. Occasionally it is useful for examination of the retina, but not before dilating the pupil.

CLINICAL SKILLS

- Measurement of visual acuity
- Testing the integrity of the visual field
- Testing pupil reactions
- Everting the upper eyelid
- Testing corneal sensation
- Fluorescein staining of the cornea
- Digital tonometry
- Testing eye movements
- Use of the ophthalmoscope.

Measurement of visual acuity

This is a test of foveal function, and each eye is tested independently. A Snellen chart, preferably an illuminated one, is placed 6 m (20 ft) from the patient and the patient is invited to read the letters. Distance glasses, if worn, should be used, although do note that patients will often put on their reading glasses when invited to 'read' the test chart. Each line on the Snellen chart has a number written below it (Figure 2.2). The acuity is noted down in two parts:

- The first number is the distance between patient and chart, usually 6 m

Figure 2.2 Snellen test chart.

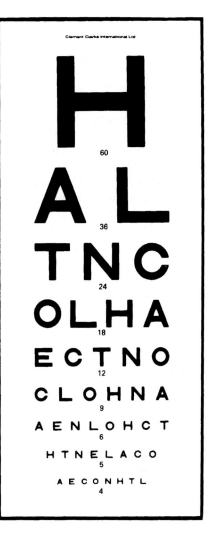

- The second number corresponds to the line on the chart with the smallest letters that the patient was able to read; 6/6 (20/20 in old money) is considered normal, although most patients can see lines of letters lower than this (e.g. 6/5).

Failure to achieve 6/60 vision is recorded as counting fingers (CF), hand movements (HM), perception of light (PL) or no perception of light (NPL), depending on what the patient can perceive.

Testing the integrity of the visual field

Confrontational visual field testing is an extremely crude test of the visual field, made even cruder by the lack of any great sensitivity in the peripheral retina (see Chapter 1). The purpose of this test is not to delineate the extent of a patient's visual field, and nor is it to compare the patient's visual field with your own (a completely pointless task that is also physically impossible, although often peddled in undergraduate textbooks). The purpose is twofold, depending on the clinical situation:

- In an asymptomatic patient we are trying to exclude any occult defect, typically bitemporal hemianopia in a patient with signs of pituitary disease.
- In a patient with visual loss we are trying to delineate the pattern of the field loss, as this is often very helpful in establishing the diagnosis. Specific patterns of field loss should be anticipated:

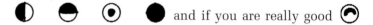 and if you are really good

Technique

Each eye should be tested independently using any convenient object of smallish size (a swab stick, hatpin, or the top of a biro pen). Imagine the patient is holding a circular tray 1 m in diameter out at arm's length; this is about the extent of the field that should be tested (Figure 2.3).

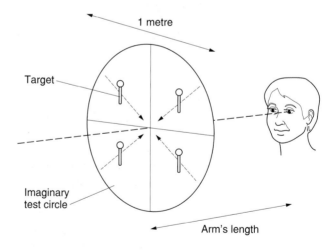

Figure 2.3 With the eye to be examined in the centre of the imaginary test circle, the target is brought in from the periphery towards the centre in each quadrant.

Testing pupil reactions

Two tests are useful; direct light reaction and the swinging light test.

Figure 2.4 Normal pupil reactions. Light on one eye causes constriction of both pupils – direct and consensual reflex.

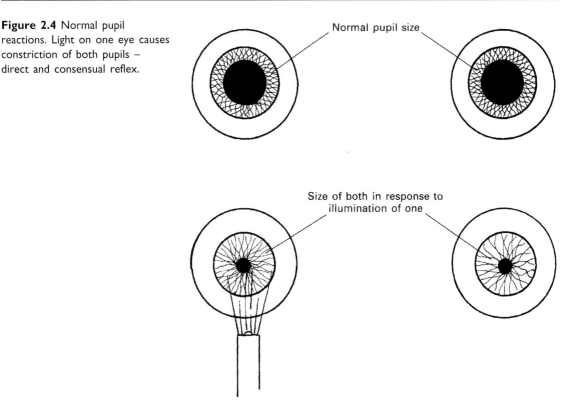

Normal pupil size

Size of both in response to illumination of one

Direct light reaction

In the direct light reaction test (Figure 2.4), no response suggests:

- A blind eye
- Pressure on the third nerve (communication of the pupillary light reflex from the midbrain to the iris is via parasympathetic nerve fibres hitchhiking with the third nerve)

    Extradural haematoma: the patient is semiconscious, 'blowing a pupil'

    Aneurysm of the circle of Willis: the patient presents with a painful third nerve palsy
- Direct trauma to the eye

    Rupture of the iris muscle, which is usually associated with a hyphaema; the patient is fully conscious
- Acute glaucoma

    The patient presents with a painful red eye with normal eye movements
- Adie pupil – a common cause of different sized pupils, especially in healthy females.

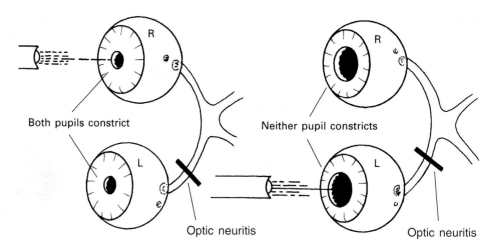

Both pupils constrict

Neither pupil constricts

Optic neuritis

Optic neuritis

Figure 2.5 A relative afferent pupillary defect. Light presented to the healthy right eye induces constriction in both pupils. On swinging the light over to the damaged eye, the pupil starts to dilate due to loss of the consensual reflex induced by previously shining the light into the healthy eye. The pupil fails to constrict normally because optic neuritis disrupts the direct pupil reflex.

The clinical situation will suggest which of the above is the cause.

The swinging light test

The swinging light test exposes reduced neuronal impulses from the retina to the optic tract, and is useful in the assessment of patients with reduced visual acuity.

To perform the test, illuminate one eye and then swing the light across the nose to illuminate the other eye. Continue this back and forth motion two or three times, dwelling on each eye long enough to induce pupillary constriction. Dilatation of either pupil when illuminated indicates reduced neuronal impulses along the optic nerve on that side, and this is called an afferent pupillary defect (Figure 2.5).

Causes include:
● A massive decrease in retinal function
    Central retinal artery occlusion
    Ischaemic central retinal vein occlusion
    A large retinal detachment
    Advanced glaucoma
● A conduction defect in the optic nerve
    Optic neuritis
    Pressure on the optic nerve.

Everting the upper lid

To evert the upper lid:
● Ask the patient to look down and grasp the lashes with the finger and thumb (Figure 2.6)
● Rotate the upper lid over the cotton bud and examine the tarsal conjunctiva for foreign bodies (Figure 2.7).

Figure 2.6 Counter-traction is best applied with a cotton bud.

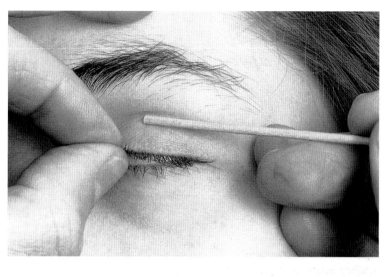

Figure 2.7 Everted upper lid.

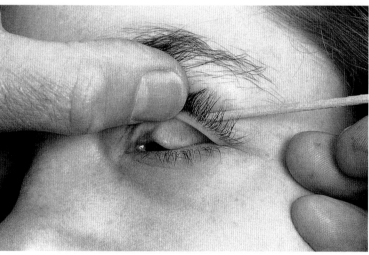

Testing corneal sensation

Roll up a piece of tissue paper into a point and, holding the lids apart, gently touch the peripheral cornea. Ask the patient if the contact with the eye could be felt. It is often useful to compare the level of sensation between the two eyes. Corneal sensation is absent during herpetic infection of the cornea.

Fluorescein staining of the cornea

Moisten the fluorescein tip with tears from the lower conjunctival sac (Figure 2.8). Orange staining of the tear film is rapid,

Figure 2.8 Applying fluorescein.

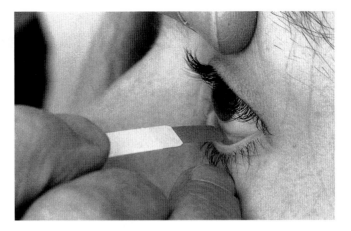

and after the patient has blinked a couple of times the dye is spread over the surface of the cornea. Fluorescein dye will stain any defects of the corneal epithelium.

Digital tonometry

Tonometry refers to the measurement of intraocular pressure, but a rough guide can be gained with the fingers. This technique is useful to exclude acute glaucoma, where the eye is rock hard due to high intraocular pressure. The normal eye is softish.

The other fingers are rested on the patient's brow, and the index fingers are used to palpate the eye alternately as if examining a skin swelling (Figure 2.9).

Figure 2.9 Digital tonometry.

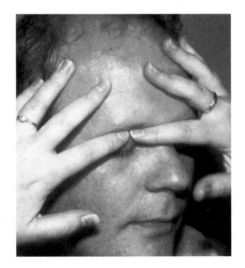

Testing eye movements

Examination of the eyes in the primary position (looking straight ahead) reveals if the eyes are squinting or not. This can be confirmed using the cover test (see Chapter 25). Testing horizontal eye movements will then expose any muscle paralysis. Abnormal movements in one eye can be the result of:

● Cranial nerve palsy
● Restriction of the eye muscles
        Inflammation
        Orbital cellulites
        Thyroid eye disease
● Mechanical damage
        Blow-out fracture.

If both eyes are abnormal, it suggests:

● Bilateral inflammatory disease – e.g. thyroid eye disease
● Problems with co-ordination of the eyes, which usually relates to brainstem disease.

The most profitable positions to test are horizontal eye movements and upgaze.

Use of the ophthalmoscope

A well-charged instrument makes an excellent torch for testing pupil reactions, and it can also be used as a magnifying glass with light source attached. To explore this possibility and to gain dexterity with the focusing wheel, hold the ophthalmoscope, with the zero lens in the eyepiece, up to your eye and examine your own fingernail from a distance of about 2 cm. You will need to move the focusing wheel to achieve a clear picture.

Retinal examination

This is all about set-up and confidence. Practice, even on your fingernail, increases the latter.

Set-up:
● Dilate the pupil with 1 per cent tropicamide.
● Ask the patient to look directly ahead and fix on an object that is at eye level. It is most important that you know that the eyes are looking straight ahead and not up or down, as this will shift the orientation of structures within the eye.

Figure 2.10 Examining the fundus. Remember to get as close as you can.

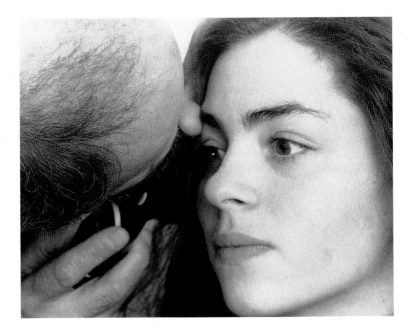

- Have the zero lens in the eyepiece and, approaching from the temporal side, come as close to the eye as possible (perhaps 2 cm; it gives an infinitely better view, honestly!). Examining from too great a distance is a common error.
- Move the focusing wheel clockwise if the instrument is in the right hand, or anticlockwise if in the left hand, until a clear view is obtained (Figure 2.10).

Confidence:
- When using the focusing wheel, don't give up; the retina will eventually come into focus with persistence, but it may take a number of turns of the wheel. The thing is not to turn one way and then the other and back again, and then give up when no view materializes. Practising looking at your fingernail at different distances will help.
- Retinal anatomy is extremely consistent. This means that the optic disc will always be found on the horizontal plane and slightly medially if the patient is looking straight ahead. To find the disc immediately, imagine a straight line that enters the eye and exits the head behind the opposite ear. If you look down this line, the disc will be there.
- The foveal area is best examined by asking the patient to look directly into the light.

Observations:
- The disc
   Note the clarity of the margin; it should be distinct

Note the colour; it should be pink

Note the cup; a large cup may indicate glaucoma

● The vessels

These can be seen to advantage using the green light on the instrument

Note variations in calibre

● The macula/fovea

Haemorrhages are also easily seen with a green light

Look for yellow, hard exudates

Look for white cotton-wool spots.

Textbook pictures

The retinal photographs in this book are taken using an indirect ophthalmoscope, which gives a wide field of view at lower magnification. The direct ophthalmoscope (the one you have got) gives a narrow field of view at high magnification, which makes it impossible to obtain an overall view. Instead, the fundus has to be seen in multiple small circular segments (Figure 2.11).

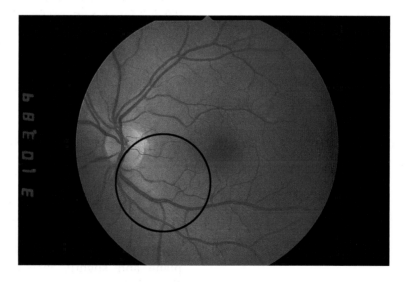

Figure 2.11 Fundal picture taken with an indirect ophthalmoscope. The inset circle is the maximum field of view obtainable with a direct ophthalmoscope.

Glasses, contact lenses and lasers

REFRACTIVE ERROR (AMETROPIA) AND ITS CORRECTION

The eye with normal vision (emmetropia) brings parallel rays of light, from objects greater than 6 m away, to a focal point on the fovea. As objects come up closer, this focal point moves behind the retina. To compensate for this, the eye accommodates (Figure 3.1). Progressive loss of distensibility of the lens with age (presbyopia) means that around the mid-forties help in the form of reading glasses is required (Figure 3.2). Some eyes do not fit this pattern due to a refractive error (ametropia).

Figure 3.1 Distance and near vision. By increasing the convexity of the crystalline lens the power in the eye is increased, and this maintains focus of the near object on the fovea.

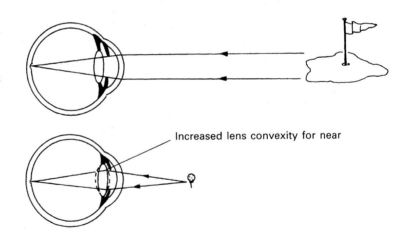

Increased lens convexity for near

Long sight (hypermetropia)

The focusing power of hypermetropic eyes is not strong enough to bring parallel rays of light onto the fovea, and instead the rays overshoot and focus behind the retina. The focusing power of these eyes can be augmented in two ways:

- By using magnifying lenses within spectacle frames
- By accommodation – low degrees of hypermetropia can be compensated for increasing the power of the eye in the

Figure 3.2 Presbyopia. The arms seem to become too short to hold the book far enough away. A magnifying lens is required to help with reading but since no lens is required for distance half-moon glasses are ideal.

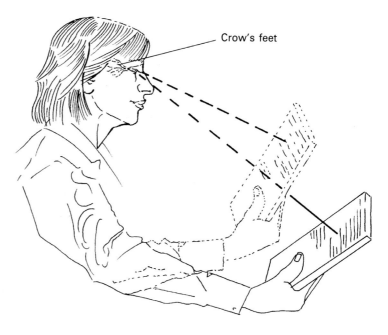

Crow's feet

Figure 3.3 The long-sighted eye. With much of the range of focus for near taken up to see in the distance, reading becomes a problem at an earlier age (perhaps in the early thirties). Patients at this stage usually revert to wearing glasses for distance, releasing accommodation to help with reading once again.

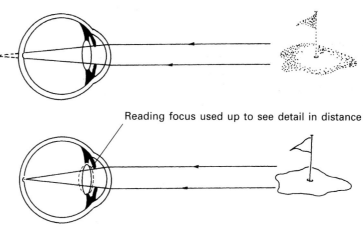

Reading focus used up to see detail in distance

same way as normal sighted eyes do for reading (Figure 3.3).

Short sight (myopia)

The focusing power of myopic eyes is too strong and parallel rays of light are brought to a focal point in the vitreous, short of the fovea (Figure 3.4). The focusing power of these eyes needs to be reduced, and only minifying lenses can do this. For near vision, however, the extra power of these eyes allows

Figure 3.4 The short-sighted eye. Minifying lenses reduce the power of the eye. If you pick up a set of minifying lenses and look through them, all objects will appear abnormally small.

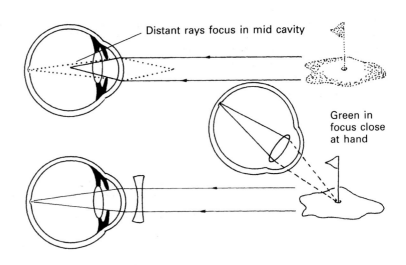

Distant rays focus in mid cavity

Green in focus close at hand

comfortable reading without glasses although most people will leave their glasses on and accommodate like the rest of us. This option is only removed when accommodative power is lost in the mid-forties. At this stage, myopes can either remove their glasses to read or they can obtain a reading correction within existing spectacles ('bifocals').

Astigmatism

To create a focal point a lens has to have a perfectly uniform curvature; non-uniform curvature would lead to more than one focal point and a blurred image. A useful analogy is to imagine a tennis ball cut in half. Lying dome-up in your palm a uniform curvature is presented; however, if you now squeeze the tennis ball into an oval shape the uniformity of curvature is lost, with one long axis and one short axis at 90° to the former being generated. If this were a lens instead of a single focal point there would now be two focal points, one for each axis, and consequently a blurred image. This situation is known as regular astigmatism (from the Greek *stigma*: point), and is relatively common in the general population although usually very mild. Astigmatism is constant throughout life unless some process affects corneal shape, such as cataract surgery or intrinsic corneal disease (e.g. keratoconus). A major driver of the popularity of phakoemulsification cataract surgery is that the technique produces negligible amounts of astigmatism postoperatively. This is due to the relatively small wound required to remove the cataract when compared with other techniques. Cylindrical lenses have the ability to change the focal point of one axis without changing the other, and thus re-establish a single point focus in astigmatic eyes.

Figure 3.5 Principle of contact lenses. The lens sits on top of the cornea, separated from it by the tear film. The front surface of the lens now becomes the main refracting surface of the eye.

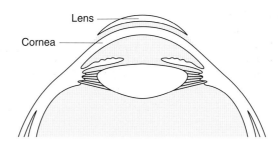

Lens

Cornea

CONTACT LENSES

As mentioned in Chapter 1, the cornea is the most powerful lens of the eye. However, if a contact lens with a different surface curvature but a similar refractive index were laid on top of the cornea, the focusing power of the eye would be altered. Contact lenses therefore merely add an extra layer to the cornea, with a back surface that parallels the corneal surface and a front surface that can be manipulated to correct most refractive errors (Figure 3.5).

Hard lenses are rigid and uncomfortable to wear. They require a period of adaptation, and not everyone can tolerate them. They are also impermeable to oxygen, and so wearing time needs to be limited to preserve corneal health.

Soft lenses are variably permeable to oxygen ('gas-permeable lenses'), and this allows extended wear in the more permeable types. They are comfortable to wear and are by far the most common lenses worn today. They are hydrophilic and so attract organisms and chemicals such as chlorine and lens cleaning solutions, and it is therefore vitally important that these lenses are cleaned correctly and that they are used precisely according to the manufacturer's directions. Failure to do this is the commonest reason for complications. Dyes such as fluorescein are also readily absorbed, so lenses should be removed before staining the cornea for examination purposes.

Complications

Complications resulting from the use of contact lenses arise from:

● Overuse, which will often present acutely as a red and painful eye; patients should be carefully examined to exclude corneal ulceration

- Overnight wear after a good party may result in pain and blepharospasm reminiscent of a corneal abrasion
- Extending the use of daily disposable lenses to 2 days instead of one for financial reasons converts a safe lens into a game of Russian roulette – corneal bacterial ulceration is always a threat
- Peripheral corneal vascularization is an indication of chronic hypoxia of the cornea due to overuse, and is normally spotted by the optician.

● A poor cleaning regimen; this can present acutely with a red and painful eye or more insidiously with an itchy eye with reduced lens tolerance

- Acute presentation may signal corneal ulceration usually with bacteria or more rarely with acanthamoeba; the latter is a common organism found in tap water, which is cheaper than lens cleaning solutions and more palatable than saliva (yes, some people lick their lenses and put them back in!)
- Reduced tolerance and discomfort following removal of the lens are typical; poor cleaning leads to deposits forming on the lens, and these act as allergens.

Action

Mild cases of discomfort can be safely referred to the dispensing optician for further advice while acute cases should be examined for evidence of corneal ulceration. Pain in the morning after overnight wear is successfully treated with chloramphenicol ointment and padding along with suitable pain relief. Resolution should occur in 24 hours if the diagnosis is correct.

LASER CORRECTION OF AMETROPIA

This has largely superseded older surgical techniques such as radial keratotomy where radial incisions in the cornea were used to flatten the centre and thus reduce myopia. Excimer lasers developed in Silicone Valley to cut microcircuit boards can accurately excise corneal tissue to an exact depth with minimal tissue damage. They are used to sculpt what is in effect a permanent contact lens onto the anterior corneal surface. There are two main methods of treatment:

● Photorefractive keratectomy (PRK)
● Laser *in-situ* keratomileusis (LASIK).

The main risk with both these techniques is a final visual acuity (with appropriate glasses) that is poorer than at the start (with appropriate glasses). This occurs in perhaps 2–3 per cent of cases. Less of a serious risk is that the treatment does not deliver 'perfect' vision without spectacles, but leaves the patient with residual amounts of myopia or hypermetropia that are correctable with a relevant prescription. Retreatment in these cases is possible. Important points for prospective patients to consider are:

- Is perfect vision required for work? (A very small number of ophthalmologists have had the procedure despite a high incidence of myopia in this group.)
- If there is significant astigmatism, the results are likely to be less successful.
- Patients should be older than 21 years, because up to that age myopia is unstable.
- Higher degrees of myopia give more unpredictable results.
- Listen carefully to the counselling given by a prospective surgeon.

Photorefractive keratectomy

Photorefractive keratectomy (PRK) is capable of treating mild to moderate degrees of myopia and mild degrees of astigmatism and hypermetropia. The procedure involves removal of the corneal epithelium with laser being applied to the underlying corneal stroma.

- Treatment time is approximately 30–60 seconds
- Postoperative pain is significant, as the corneal epithelium is scraped off and will take 2–3 days to heal
- Corneal haze develops in 2 weeks (Figure 3.6), can persist for some months, and in some cases permanently reduces the visual acuity
- Ninety per cent of cases will have reasonable vision without spectacles.

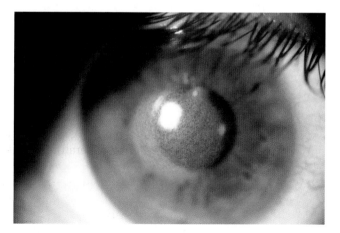

Figure 3.6 Corneal haze. If this does not dissipate, visual acuity will suffer. Reproduced with permission from *Clinical Ophthalmology* by J. Kanski, 1999.

Laser *in-situ* keratomileusis

Laser *in-situ* keratomileusis (LASIK) is capable of treating higher degrees of myopia, and has the advantages of speedier

Figure 3.7 Laser *in-situ* keratomileusis (LASIK). A corneal flap has been raised prior to laser. Reproduced with permission from *Clinical Ophthalmology* by J. Kanski, 1999.

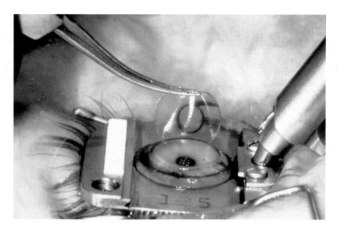

visual rehabilitation and no postoperative pain. The technique involves creating a corneal flap with a microkeratome (Figure 3.7) and lasering the underlying stroma, followed by replacement of the flap (hence the term 'flap and zap').

OTHER METHODS OF CORRECTING AMETROPIA

Laser techniques concentrate on altering the shape of the cornea, but other methods have been developed that manipulate the power of the crystalline lens:

Intraocular lenses may be used in two ways:

- Removal of a normal crystalline lens and replacement with an appropriate intraocular implant in a manner similar to a cataract extraction
- Intraocular lenses that sit on top of the crystalline lens.

These methods are practised in some areas, but run the rare risk of intraocular infection (endophthalmitis) and cataract formation in the case of the latter.

In summary, some of the methods described above are very successful and many patients are very happy with the results; however, all methods carry a risk to visual acuity and prospective patients should be aware of these risks and carefully weigh them up against the potential benefits of 'normal sight'.

Part 1

Visual disturbance

4

Introduction to visual disturbance

The whole purpose of the eye is vision, so it is not surprising that complaints about visual disturbance are common. Since vision is so vital to normal life patients are often very anxious, but none the less a detailed account of the complaint is vital. The main visual disturbances and common causes are:

● Sudden loss of vision
    Vein/artery occlusions
    Macular haemorrhage
    Retinal detachment
    Ocular migraine
    Amaurosis fugax
● Sudden blurring of vision
    Central serous retinopathy
    Mild vein occlusion
● Gradual blurring of vision
    Cataract
    Age-related macular degeneration
● Distorted vision
    Macular degeneration
    Macular hole
    Cellophane maculopathy
● Flashes and floaters
    Posterior vitreous detachment
    Vitreous haemorrhage
    Migraine
● Double vision
    Blow-out fracture
    Cranial nerve palsy.

Sudden loss of vision

Don't panic! In these cases there is nothing that can usefully be done to bring vision back. However, all cases will require referral to the eye department; the key is to decide how urgently. Two causes require urgent referral:

- Giant cell arteritis (temporal arteritis) – immediate treatment protects the other eye from the same fate
- Retinal detachment – vision can be restored with timely intervention.

Giant cell arteritis (temporal arteritis)

This is a rare condition that is most prevalent in the seventh and eighth decades. It is an inflammatory reaction against elastin in the walls of arteries. The arteries of the scalp, including the temporal artery, and the arteries supplying the eye are rich in elastin and so are commonly affected. The retina and optic nerve are supplied with blood by the central retinal artery, but an anatomical idiosyncrasy means that the posterior ciliary artery supplies the head of the optic nerve, including the optic disc. While giant cell arteritis can affect both these arteries, the posterior ciliaries are particularly susceptible. Occlusion of an affected artery leads to infarction of the areas it supplied with blood:

- The posterior ciliary artery supplies the optic nerve head; occlusion causes 'anterior ischaemic optic neuropathy' (AION)
- The central retinal artery supplies the retina; occlusion causes 'central retinal artery occlusion' (CRAO).

If temporal arteritis remains untreated after visual loss in one eye, the other eye will be affected over the next 1–2 weeks, resulting in total blindness.

The condition is a true ophthalmic emergency, and treatment should occur if there is suspicion of the diagnosis. Confirmation of the diagnosis by temporal artery biopsy can wait. Tragic cases occasionally occur where doctors procrastinate over the diagnosis, only for it to be confirmed with the loss of vision in the remaining eye. Therefore all cases of visual loss in the relevant age group should have the diagnosis actively excluded by looking for any of the features of arteritis listed below:

- Age over 60 years
- Temporal/generalized headache
- Pain on chewing or talking (jaw claudication)
- Erythrocyte sedimentation rate over 60 mm/h
- Systemic upset – malaise, weight loss, anorexia, low-grade fever
- Psychosis (rarely).

Treatment

- Intravenous methylprednisolone 1 g/day for 3 days
- Oral prednisolone 80 mg daily.

Treatment is then tailed down to a maintenance dose, typically 10 mg prednisolone daily. The precise dose is titrated according to the level of the ESR. Treatment is often necessary for some years, and measures to guard against corticosteroid-induced osteoporosis are indicated.

INVESTIGATING SUDDEN LOSS OF VISION

History

Visual loss can be permanent or transitory, bilateral or unilateral, involve the whole visual field or only part of the field, and be associated with other clinical features such as pain or floaters. These points in the history will help to narrow the diagnostic field considerably. Particular inquiry into symptoms of temporal arteritis in cases of unilateral visual loss will guard against missing this important diagnosis.

Examination

The examination will focus on the assessment of:

- Visual acuity
- Visual field
- Red reflex
- Pupil reactions
- Fundal examination.

The visual acuity is usually severely reduced; if not, patients complain of sudden blurring rather than visual loss. Examination of the visual field will confirm the pattern of loss that they describe. In the case of hemianopia/quadrantinopia, be aware that patients may not realize that both eyes are affected; to them half of their visual field is missing and the eye that corresponds to that side is blamed for being defective. Fundal examination should only be attempted after dilating the pupil with tropicamide, as this massively enhances the view. Dilating drops should only be instilled after the pupil reactions have been tested. If a red reflex cannot be obtained, then an opacity obscuring the retinal reflex (e.g. a vitreous haemorrhage) is inferred.

Diagnosis

The flowchart in Figure 5.1 can be used to assist in identifying the cause of sudden loss of vision.

Figure 5.1 Identifying the causes of sudden loss of vision. The icons indicate the associated patterns of field loss found.

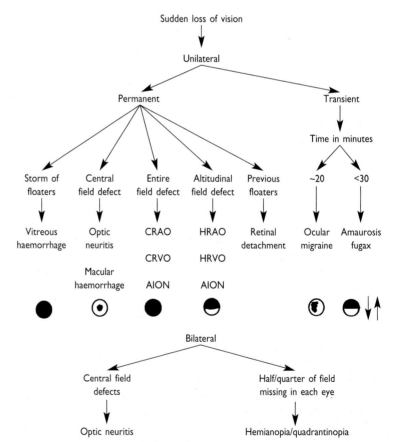

UNILATERAL PERMANENT VISUAL LOSS

Retinal detachment

The retina, like wallpaper, can fall off. Initially a tear develops in the peripheral retina, and then the retina gradually peels off, steadily moving towards the macula at the centre of the eye (Figure 5.2). Patients may report a 'dark curtain' coming across the peripheral vision, but many do not. Once the macular area is stripped off, the patient perceives a sudden loss of vision.

Figure 5.2 The advancing front of the detached retina is approaching the optic disc and macula.

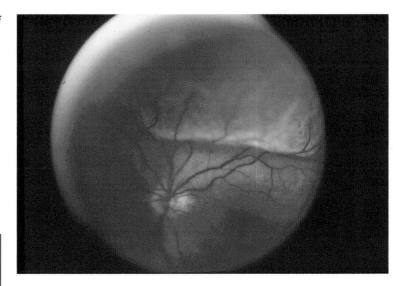

Findings

- A relative afferent pupillary defect (RAPD) will be present.
- Once the fovea is involved, central acuity drops to 6/60 or worse
- Variable field loss – this can take on any pattern
- Detached grey retina on fundal examination.

Retinal detachment can occur at any age, but is unusual below the age of 20 years. Myopia and eye trauma (including eye operations) can cause retinal holes and thus retinal detachment (see Chapter 9 for a further description of retinal hole formation). At the time of retinal hole formation most patients will complain of flashes and floaters, but it may be some days before loss of vision occurs.

Action

This symptom complex should prompt urgent referral. Reattachment is achieved by 'gluing' the retina back to the eye wall. To achieve this, the retina and the eye wall must be in apposition with some kind of 'glue' in between. The 'glue' is scarring, and this is induced either by external cryotherapy or internal laser. The eye wall and the retina are opposed either by use of an external buckle (Figure 5.3) or by inserting a gas bubble (Figure 5.4). Recovery of vision is often reasonable provided surgery occurs within a day or so of detachment. Postoperatively, corticosteroid drops QID and dilating drops are typically used for 2–3 months.

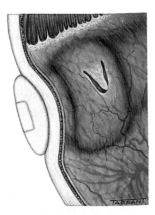

Figure 5.3 The buckle indents the eye wall so that it becomes apposed to the retina. Prior cryotherapy in the area induces scar formation, which closes the hole. Reproduced with permission from *Clinical Ophthalmology* by J. Kanski, 1999.

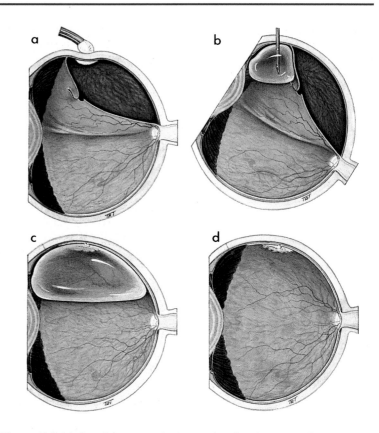

Figure 5.4 (a) Cryotherapy to the external wall induces scar formation. (b) and (c) Injection of a gas bubble tamponades the retina against the eye wall. (d) Sealing of the retinal hole by scar formation.

Vitreous haemorrhage

Visual loss associated with a coincident storm of floaters is indicative of a vitreous haemorrhage. These occur as the result of rupture of new vessels in diabetic retinopathy, but in the absence of diabetes they indicate avulsion of a retinal blood vessel secondary to vitreous traction (see Chapter 9). A retinal hole has also more than likely developed, and the patient should be under the close observation of the eye department to monitor the situation as the haemorrhage clears.

Findings

- Normal pupil reaction.
- No red reflex. This is absent as the blood in the vitreous obscures the reflection of the retina's red glow.

Retinal artery occlusion

This condition causes sudden permanent loss of vision in the retinal area affected. It is embolic or thrombotic in origin, and

Figure 5.5 Central retinal artery occlusion. The whole retina is infracted and oedematous, like a giant cotton-wool spot. The thin retina at the fovea allows a red glow from the unaffected choroidal circulation to show through.

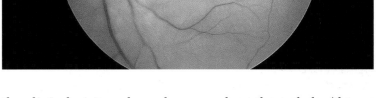

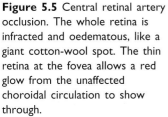

the clinical picture depends upon where the embolus/thrombus eventually sticks:

- Central retinal artery (Figure 5.5) – total visual field defect [●]
- Branch of CRA (Figure 5.6) – altitudinal field defect (top or bottom half only) [○].

Of the two, central retinal artery occlusion is the commonest. The classic 'cherry-red spot' shown in Figure 5.5 only lasts for a few hours, after which time the oedema caused by infracted retina starts to settle. Thereafter the retinal appearance can look surprisingly normal. (Incidentally, the 'cherry-red spot' represents a view of the underlying choroidal blood

Figure 5.6 An embolus blocking the superior branch of the central retinal artery can be seen. Only the top half of the retina is oedematous.

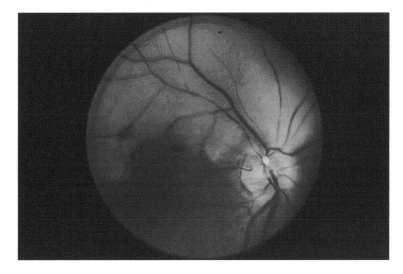

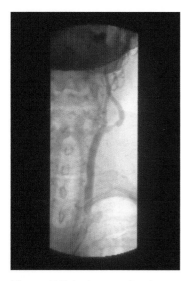

Figure 5.7 Angiogram showing significant stenosis of the internal carotid artery.

through the thin foveal retina, while the rest of the choroidal circulation is obscured by oedematous and infarcted retina.) Branch retinal artery occlusions are embolic in origin, and cholesterol or calcific emboli can often be seen trapped in the bore of the blood vessel. Vision does not return to the infarcted retina, but if the fovea is spared central acuity may be retained. The visual prognosis for the eye as a whole is good if the macula is spared, but visual field loss in the affected area is permanent.

Findings

- RAPD present
- Visual acuity if the fovea is affected will be very poor (< 6/60)
- Field assessment will confirm the pattern of the defect, and shows total loss or altitudinal defects
- Cherry-red spot on fundal examination; fundal examination may show white, fluffy, oedematous retina, and perhaps an obvious embolus
- Auscultation of neck – search for a carotid bruit
- Exclude temporal arteritis.

Action

The ophthalmic artery, from which the central retinal artery derives, is the first branch of the internal carotid. The second branch is the middle cerebral artery, which supplies most of the brain. Therefore, patients who experience embolic phenomena in the eye are at risk of future emboli causing a cerebral infarct or stroke. With this in mind a full cardiovascular examination is indicated, including auscultation of the neck in search of a carotid bruit. Patients should also be referred for duplex scanning of the carotid arteries (Figure 5.7). If significant stenosis is found, carotid endarterectomy may be indicated to prevent future strokes. If not, aspirin 75 mg daily is effective.

Findings

- RAPD
- Field assessment shows total loss or altitudinal defects (top or bottom half; this is suggestive of non-arteritic AION)
- Swollen, pale (infracted) optic disc on fundal examination, often with overlying flame haemorrhabes (Figure 5.8)
- Giant cell arteritis should be actively excluded, as AION is its commonest ocular presentation.

Anterior ischaemic optic neuropathy

In anterior ischaemic optic neuropathy (AION) the blood supply (posterior ciliary arteries) to the optic nerve head and disc is cut off, causing infarction. The cause can be arteritic (temporal arteritis) or non-arteritic (embolic). The prognosis for visual improvement in the affected eye is poor.

Action

- Arteritic – immediate corticosteroid treatment
- Nonarteritic – as for retinal artery occlusion

Figure 5.8 The disc is swollen and pale, reflecting infarction of the nerve head. Dilated capillaries running over the nerve head, giving a much redder appearance, typify other types of disc oedema.

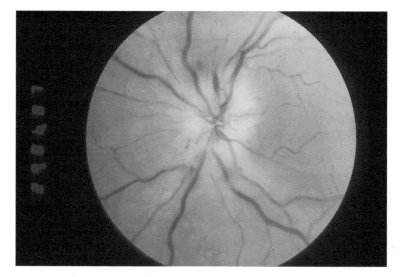

Retinal vein occlusion

With retinal vein occlusion, the degree of visual acuity loss is variable and some patients may only complain of visual blurring. This condition is associated with hypertension, diabetes, smoking and glaucoma. It is a common cause of sudden visual loss. As in CRAO, different field defects occur depending the part of the vein affected:

- Central retinal vein (Figure 5.9) – total visual field defect
- Branch of CRV (Figure 5.10) – altitudinal field defect (top or bottom half only).

Figure 5.9 Central retinal vein occlusion. The haemorrhage is within the nerve fibre layer and thus often gives an impression of the organization of nerve fibres in the retina (see Figure 1.5).

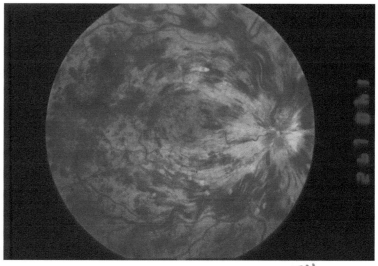

Figure 5.10 Branch retinal vein occlusion. This only affects the top or bottom half of the retina, but the underlying pathology is the same as that of central retinal vein occlusions.

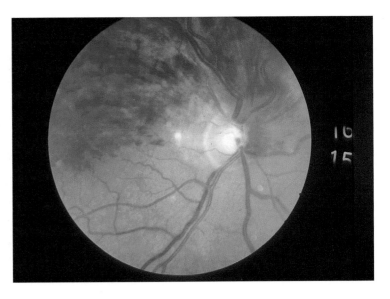

Findings

- RAPD present
- Field assessment shows total loss or altitudinal defects
- 'Stormy sunset' fundal appearance.

Action

Referral is not urgent, but these patients do require follow-up within I month. Profound retinal ischaemia induces the formation of new blood vessels on the optic disc or on the iris (see Chapter 22). These can have severe complications such as secondary glaucoma and possible loss of the eye. If this situation occurs, laser therapy is helpful. Visual recovery is variable. In up to 10 per cent of cases the other eye suffers a vein occlusion later. Associated hypertension should be treated.

Macular haemorrhage

Macular degeneration is the commonest reason for blindness in the western world. Eighty per cent of cases are associated with a gradual degeneration in macular function (see Chapter 7); however, in 20 per cent of patients a subretinal neovascular membrane develops. This can suddenly bleed, causing a macular haemorrhage with central visual field loss (Figure 5.11).

Findings

- Poor visual acuity with central field loss only
- Normal pupil reactions
- Fundoscopy reveals haemorrhage over the macular area.

Action

Urgent review of these cases is required because a corresponding neovascular membrane can be present in the other eye, and some of these are occasionally treatable with laser. The visual prognosis for the affected eye is poor, as macular scarring follows resolution of the haemorrhage.

Figure 5.11 Severe macular haemorrhage. There is blood covering most of the macula area.

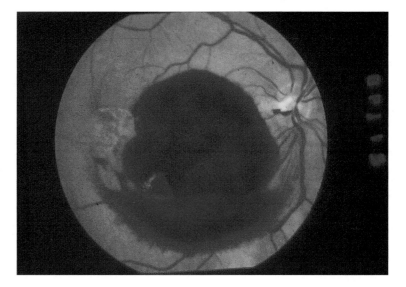

Laser treatment

A combination of specialist clinical examination and fluorescein angiography of the other eye may reveal the presence of a subretinal neovascular membrane (Figure 5.12). Lasers can be used to destroy these new vessels, but it must be remembered that laser therapy is destructive and surrounding retina will also be destroyed as part of the treatment process. Up until recently this meant that neovascular membranes under the fovea were untreatable because of collateral damage to the fovea caused by the laser treatment.

Figure 5.12 Picture of a fluorescein angiogram showing a lacy pattern of subretinal neovascular membrane. If this is left untreated bleeding will eventually occur, with loss of central visual acuity. Reproduced with permission from *Clinical Ophthalmology* by J. Kanski, 1999.

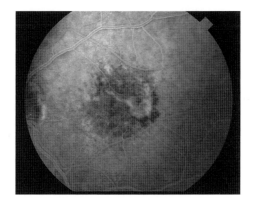

Photodynamic therapy

Photodynamic therapy (PDT) is a new treatment for the destruction of subretinal neovascular membranes that has proven benefit in particular cases. Although this treatment modality still uses lasers, the target blood vessels are first sensitized by a light-sensitive drug. This allows precise destruction of the blood vessels without damage to the fovea and macula.

Optic neuritis

This condition is usually unilateral and mainly affects younger patients between the ages of 20 and 50 years, although any age can be affected. The majority of cases are due to a demyelinating episode, although some cases follow a viral illness. The presentation is typical and involves sudden loss of central vision associated with vague aching pain behind or in the eye, which is exacerbated by eye movement.

Usually inflammation affects the mid-section of the nerve ('retrobulbar neuritis'), but occasionally inflammation affects the anterior portion of the nerve, in which case the disc becomes swollen (Figure 5.13). Visual acuity usually recovers within 4–6 weeks, but vision often deteriorates further in the days following initial presentation.

Findings

- Typical history – a decrease in colour vision (especially for red) and a central field defect are typical
- RAPD is present
- Normal fundus/papillitis.

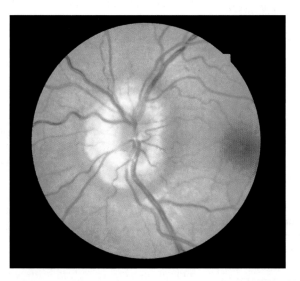

Figure 5.13 'Papillitis'. This can be differentiated from AION on the basis of the patient's young age and history of an aching eye. Papilloedema is discounted because it is bilateral and does not cause visual loss.

Action

Young patients are very anxious and need to be reassured that their vision will return in a few weeks. At the same time, patients need to be told that their vision is likely to worsen in the coming few days. Severe and bilateral cases can be given high-dose intravenous and oral corticosteroids to speed up recovery time. The final visual acuity is not, however, affected, and this treatment is therefore not given in routine cases.

Association with multiple sclerosis

Approximately 70 per cent of women and 35 per cent of men will ultimately develop other neurological problems and be diagnosed as having multiple sclerosis.

UNILATERAL TRANSIENT LOSS OF VISION

Amaurosis fugax

> **Action**
>
> Patients are at substantial risk of cerebral stroke, and should be placed on aspirin as well as being referred to the vascular surgeons for duplex carotid scanning.

This a transient ischaemic attack affecting the retina. It is embolic in origin, and patients describe a typical history of a 'curtain' that falls across the vision, remains for 2–3 minutes and then lifts. The fundus is normal and visual prognosis is good.

Ocular migraine

> **Findings**
>
> • Typical history especially duration of visual loss differentiates these two diagnoses.

Patients complain of missing patches in the vision associated with flashes, quivering or scintillating lights. Symptoms typically last 20 minutes, with normal vision restored after this period. There is no history of headache. No treatment is required apart from reassurance.

BILATERAL LOSS OF VISION

Homonymous hemianopia and quadrantinopia

> **Action**
>
> Aspirin treatment can prevent further recurrences. Patients should be advised to stop driving, as hemianopia does not satisfy the legal requirement for driving (see Chapter 28).

Patients complain of sudden loss of half of their vision. Visual acuity is usually good, but there is loss of half the visual field in each eye. No other symptoms occur. The cause is an occlusion of one of the posterior cerebral arteries. These arteries supply the left and right occipital cortices. Each occipital cortex deals with information for one half of the visual field. This information is gathered by both eyes, but ends up going to one side or other by virtue of relevant nerve fibres crossing in the optic chiasm. The macular area and hence central visual acuity is spared because the middle cerebral artery supplies this particular area of the visual cortex. The field defect usually improves over the next 4–8 weeks.

Typical visual field loss

Sudden blurring of vision

The severity of visual loss in conditions such as central retinal vein occlusion, optic neuritis and macular haemorrhage can vary. Severe visual loss will be perceived as a sudden loss of vision, while in less severe cases patients may complain of sudden blurring of vision. Conditions that may cause this include:

- Central retinal vein occlusion
- Optic neuritis
- Macular haemorrhage
- Central serous retinopathy
- Posterior uveitis.

Visual acuity is only moderately reduced (6/12–6/18), and this makes visual field assessment rather difficult. Patients with optic neuritis will have a subtle afferent pupillary defect, while the fundal appearances of CRVO (Figure 6.1) and macular haemorrhage (Figure 6.2) are essentially the same but less marked (see Chapter 5).

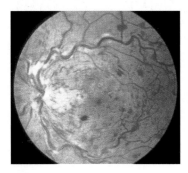

Figure 6.1 Central retinal vein occlusion. Vision is moderately reduced due to associated macular oedema.

Figure 6.2 Macular haemorrhage. Blood surrounds the foveal area.

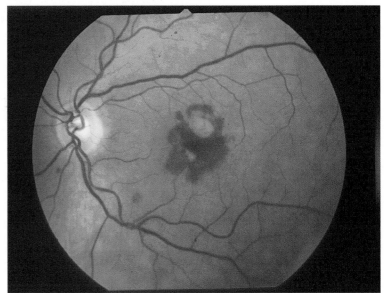

CENTRAL SEROUS RETINOPATHY

This predominantly affects young or middle-aged men, although women of the same age group are also occasionally affected. Central visual acuity is suddenly reduced to approximately 6/12, due to fluid leaking under the retina of the macular area.

Findings

The eye appears normal, but under binocular indirect ophthalmoscopy a slight round swelling of the macula is evident (Figure 6.3). This is very difficult to detect with an ordinary ophthalmoscope. The diagnosis can be confirmed by fluorescein angiography.

Action

An urgent outpatient appointment is indicated to confirm the diagnosis. Patients recover normal vision in a few weeks or months, but some do require laser treatment to achieve this. The condition is occasionally recurrent.

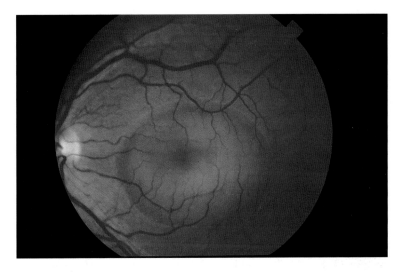

Figure 6.3 Central serous retinopathy. A faint oval shape is seen surrounding the fovea. Reproduced with permission from *Clinical Ophthalmology* by J. Kanski, 1999.

Gradual blurring of vision

Most patients with gradual blurring of vision will do the obvious thing and consult their optician. Many of the diagnoses in this section are brought to the attention of the doctor via an optician's letter. The common causes are generally, but not always, age related:

● Cataract
● Age-related macular degeneration
● Posterior capsular opacification (post cataract surgery).

Amongst young and middle-aged patients, blurring of vision often simply requires prescription of glasses either for distance or for reading. However, gradual visual loss may rarely be due to compression of the optic nerve by tumour – pituitary adenoma or meningioma.

  The local optician is a very helpful ally in diagnosing cases of gradual blurring of vision.

CATARACT

Increasing age is the cause of cataracts in over 90 per cent of cases. However, occasionally they occur for different reasons:

● Congenital
● Metabolic
        Diabetes (increased incidence and earlier onset)
        Corticosteroid use
● Trauma (including intraocular operations!)
● Chronic uveitis.

Types of cataract

There are several types of cataract, but two deserve special mention: nuclear sclerosis and posterior subcapsular cataract.

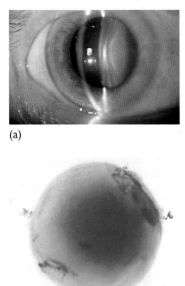

(a)

(b)

Figure 7.1 (a) Nuclear sclerosis. A slit beam of light cutting across the anterior segment of the eye highlights the brown pigment in the lens. (b) A nuclear sclerotic lens after removal from the eye. Note the density of brown pigment in the centre of the lens.

Figure 7.2 Posterior subcapsular cataract. The slit beam highlights a small area of posterior subcapsular capsule blistering against the red reflex.

Nuclear sclerosis

This is the commonest type of cataract, and is in effect an exaggeration of the normal ageing process. With increasing age the lens becomes denser and there is build up of a brown pigment (Figure 7.1). The power of the lens increases with increasing density, making patients progressively short sighted ('myopic shift') so that they require periodic visits to the optician for stronger glasses to restore visual acuity. In most cases vision gradually decreases and the patient's lifestyle is hampered quite early on.

Some patients, however, retain quite good visual acuity despite very dense brown nuclear sclerotic cataracts; a situation akin to a normal person wearing deeply tinted sunglasses. However, once these patients have one cataract removed, they become very aware of the difference in quality of vision between the two eyes and are keen for the second eye to be operated on as well.

Posterior subcapsular cataract

In this cataract a small amount of blistering of the posterior lens near to the posterior capsule causes major disruption of vision, as this is the point where light rays entering the eye cross over (Figure 7.2). In the early stages patients can maintain reasonable visual acuity, but are very troubled with symptoms such as glare.

This type of cataract is particularly associated with previous ingestion of corticosteriods.

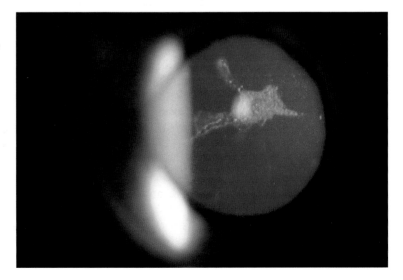

Figure 7.3 Cataract in the lens is highlighted against the red reflex.

Symptoms of cataract

- The most common is reduction in visual acuity
- Glare from the sun or oncoming traffic lights is also a common feature
- Monocular diplopia (i.e. double vision with only one eye open) is an occasional complaint.

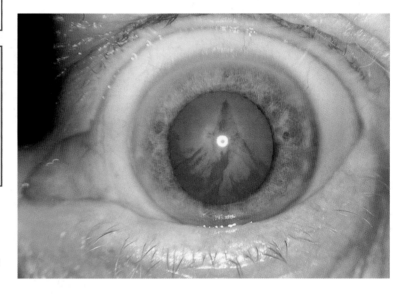

Cataract surgery

The principle is to remove the cloudy lens and then correct for the loss of its power. There are two methods:

- *Aphakic* (from the Greek *phakos*: lens). In this situation the eye is left with no lens, and thick glasses are then required to compensate for the loss of power within the eye (this method is still common in the Third World). This method gives a poor optical result and hence in the developed world it has been superseded by lens implantation. Alternatively strong contact lenses can be worn, but this is not always practical for older patients, and without their lenses in they are blind.
- *Pseudophakic.* In this situation an intraocular lens (IOL) is implanted within the eye. Sir Harold Ridley, a British ophthalmologist during the Second World War, observed a Hurricane pilot who had fragments of Perspex from the windscreen of his plane in his eye. The inertness of the Perspex gave him the idea of using Perspex to make a lens

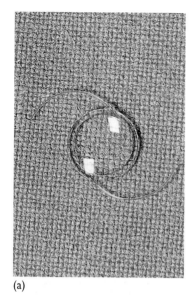

(a)

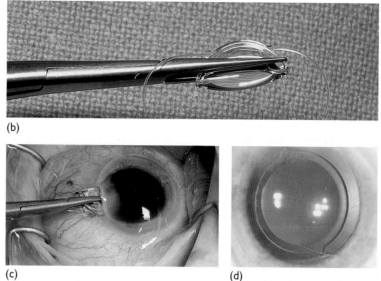

(b)

(c)   (d)

Figure 7.4 (a) Silicone foldable lens. (b) Lens folded in half. (c) Insertion of lens through a small corneal wound. (d) The lens unfolded within the eye.

for implantation after cataract removal. This idea has revolutionized modern cataract surgery. Two basic types of lens exist:

Rigid Perspex lenses, which require a larger wound to fit them into the eye

Soft foldable lenses made from silicone or acrylic, which can be folded in half and inserted into the eye where they are allowed to unfold to their natural size (Figure 7.4).

Basic techniques of cataract removal

- *Intracapsular technique.* In this technique the lens and lens capsule are removed without lens implantation.

    It results in a large wound with sutures required to close the wound, inducing higher astigmatism

    There is a high complication rate

    The patient is left aphakic.

- *Extracapsular technique.* With this method the lens is removed in one piece through a large wound and an implant is placed in the capsular bag (Figure 7.5).

    It results in a large wound with sutures required to close the wound, inducing higher astigmatism

    There is a 3-month postoperative recovery time.

- *Phakoemulsification.* Here, the lens is removed *in situ* through a small wound utilizing an ultrasound probe (Figure 7.6). A foldable implant is then placed in the capsular bag.

This results in a small wound with no suture required for closure, inducing minimal astigmatism as the original corneal shape is maintained

There is a 2-week postoperative recovery time.

Figure 7.5 A diagram demonstrating the placement of an intraocular lens within the remaining lens capsule ('capsular bag') once the cataract has been removed. The posterior lens capsule prevents the IOL from floating into the vitreous.

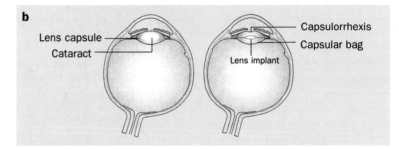

Figure 7.6 Phakoemulsification probe within the eye. The wound need only be the size of the probe, as the cataract is removed *in situ* and the IOL can be folded to slip inside the same small wound.

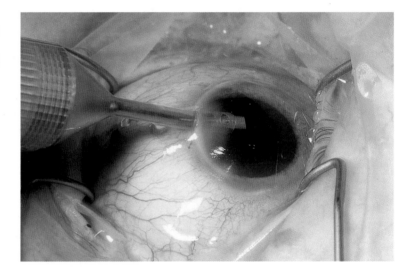

Although the first two techniques are still used for particular cases, most cases of cataract today are removed using phakoemulsification to maximize the benefits of minimal astigmatism and fast recovery time.

The cataract process

- Biometry and pre-assessment is carried out. In many units this will occur some weeks before surgery. The patient is counselled, and various measurements are taken of the eye so that a bespoke implant of appropriate power can be chosen for the patient.

- Surgery is performed. In most units this will be as a day case under local anaesthetic, which may vary from a full regional block to topical anaesthetic drops alone. General anaesthesia is also occasionally utilized in selected patients.
- Postoperative treatment is prescribed. Patients are usually treated with a combination of corticosteroid and antibiotic drops four times a day. A postoperative visit in 2–3 weeks is standard, and drop treatment is generally stopped at this point. Some units will also see patients the day after surgery. Patients who have had small incision phakoemulsification cataract surgery need only refrain from heavy lifting in the immediate postoperative period.
- An optician's visit is arranged at about 5 weeks postoperation to obtain suitable distance and reading glasses.

Complications of cataract surgery

Early

- *Posterior capsular rupture.* The capsule is only 2 μm thick and it is easily torn. Capsular rupture occurs in 1–3 per cent of cases. Support for the IOL may be compromised, and this may need to be positioned elsewhere (such as on top of the iris). If rupture occurs before all the cataract has been removed, some lens fragments may fall into the vitreous cavity. These cannot be left, as they will cause a vigorous uveitis.
- *Lens fragments in the vitreous.* In these cases, a second operation (vitrectomy) is required to remove the fragments. Although posterior capsular rupture and loss of lens fragments into the vitreous increases the likelihood of a poor outcome, most patients still achieve good postoperative visual acuity.
- *Endophthalmitis.* This is widespread bacterial infection within the eye. It occurs once in every thousand cases of cataract, although it can occur after any type of intraocular surgery. An increasingly red and painful eye in the first few days to a week after intraocular surgery is very suggestive of endophthalmitis, and requires immediate referral. After cataract surgery pain should decrease and vision should increase every day. It is a very worrying sign if either is getting worse, and this situation demands immediate referral. Up to 50 per cent of cases will have a poor outcome despite treatment.

Late

- *Retinal detachment.* Although still rare, there is an increase in the incidence after cataract surgery. Symptoms

Figure 7.7 Posterior capsular opacification. Regrowth of lens epithelial cells across the posterior capsule disrupts the normally clear red reflex.

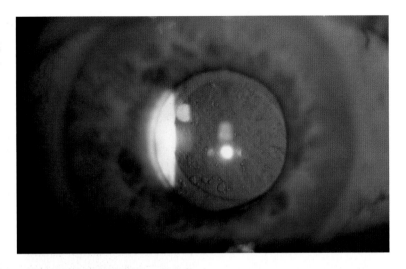

Figure 7.8 Posterior capsulotomy. The YAG laser can be used to photo-disrupt the posterior capsule, re-establishing a clear red reflex and normal vision for the patient.

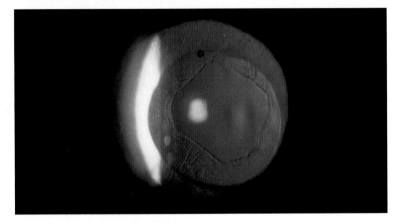

Findings
• Decreased visual acuity • Abnormal red reflex (Figure 7.7).

Action
Refer patient to the local eye hospital for YAG laser treatment (Figure 7.8). After successful capsulotomy, regrowth of lens cells does not occur. The procedure is quick and painless.

of flashes and floaters deserve referral for retinal examination.

● *Posterior capsule opacification.* Following cataract surgery, regrowth of any remaining microscopic lens epithelial cells across the posterior capsule can cause clouding of the vision. Symptoms of a gradual decrease in visual acuity some 6 months–2 years following cataract surgery are very suggestive of posterior capsule opacification.

AGE-RELATED MACULAR DEGENERATION

Macular degeneration is the most common reason for patients in the UK to be registered blind. Only the macular area is affected, and so patients retain good peripheral vision and often navigate around obstacles with apparent ease. Affected patients, who are usually in their seventies or older, complain of poor reading vision and distortion of straight lines.

Findings

- Early fundal signs are macular drusen (Figure 7.9)
- Over the coming months and years atrophy and pigmentation occur, associated with a drop in visual acuity to around 6/60 (Figure 7.10)
- Some 20 per cent of patients with macula degeneration will develop a subretinal neovascular membrane, and this can lead to sudden macular haemorrhage (see Chapter 5).

Action

There is no treatment for patients with atrophic-type macular degeneration. However, patients with sudden macular haemorrhage may harbour lesions in the fellow eye that are amenable to laser treatment (see Chapter 5).

Figure 7.9 Macular drusen. These appear as yellow lumps and represent areas of worn out retina. Reproduced with permission from *Clinical Ophthalmology* by J. Kanski, 1999.

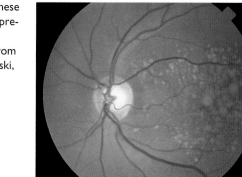

Figure 7.10 Geographic atrophy of the fovea and macula. Reproduced with permission from *Clinical Ophthalmology* by J. Kanski, 1999.

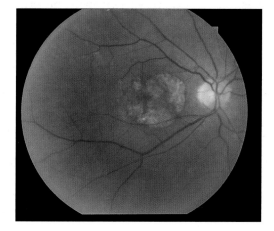

Findings

• Bitemporal hemianopia
• Headache
• Pale optic discs.

Action

Referral to an ophthalmologist to confirm possible field defects may be appropriate, but ultimately these patients require the services of a neurosurgeon.

TUMOUR

Compression of the optic nerve or optic chiasm by a tumour is a very rare cause of gradual visual failure. Pituitary adenomas in young to middle-aged adults and meningiomas in middle-aged women are the commonest culprits.

Chiasmal syndrome

Pituitary tumours pressing on the chiasm produce a classic bitemporal visual field defect (Figure 7.11). The chiasm lies a full centimetre from the normal pituitary gland and so tumours need to be of some size to produce effects on the visual field. This means that tumours producing a chiasmal syndrome do not usually produce hormones, or if they do the effects are subtle (e.g. prolactin in men – gynaecomastia, impotence). Tumours producing more obvious hormonal effects, such as amenorrhoea (prolactin in women), acromegaly (growth hormone) or Cushing's syndrome (corticotrophic hormone) are usually detected early at the microadenoma stage. These tumours do not become big enough to produce field defects.

Pressure on the dura caused by an expanding tumour means that 50 per cent of patients with tumours causing chiasmal syndrome will complain of headache.

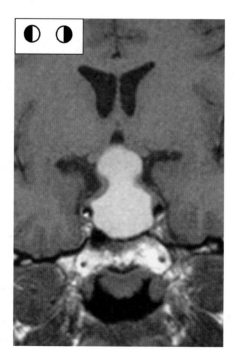

Figure 7.11 MRI scan showing a pituitary tumour that has broken through the dura covering the pituitary fossa and is pressing against the optic chiasm superiorly. Inset is the typical appearance of a bitemporal hemianopic field defect.

Distorted vision

Distortion of the vision is typical of macular disease. Patients may complain of objects being larger or smaller than they should be, or of distortion of straight lines. Causes are:

- Macular degeneration – the commonest cause (see Chapter 7)
- Macular hole
- Macular pucker.

MACULAR HOLE

This is a relatively rare kind of age-related macular degeneration, in which vitreous traction on the fovea causes a macular cyst with distortion and blurring of vision. This progresses over many months to avulsion of foveal retina causing a retinal hole (Figure 8.1). Vision is reduced to around 6/60. Fortunately, only about 10 per cent of cases are bilateral.

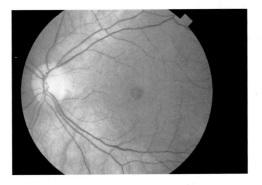

Figure 8.1 Macular hole. There is a round, punched-out missing area of retina over the fovea.
Reproduced with permission from *Clinical Ophthalmology* by J. Kanski, 1999.

During the evolution of a macular hole vitrectomy can relieve vitreous traction, but this is a high-risk procedure and results are variable. Once holes are fully formed, they are untreatable.

MACULAR PUCKER (CELLOPHANE MACULOPATHY)

Macular pucker usually occurs in late middle age. A fibrous membrane develops above the retina, and contraction of this

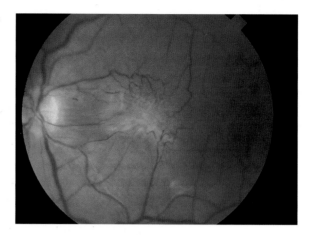

Figure 8.2 Macular pucker. There is distortion of the retina by fibrotic membranes over the fovea. Note the straightening of retinal blood vessels. Reproduced with permission from *Clinical Ophthalmology* by J. Kanski, 1999.

membrane causes subtle wrinkles in the retina, with associated distorted vision (Figuer 8.2). Detection of this condition is very difficult with a direct ophthalmoscope.

Vitrectomy segmentation of the membrane can relieve symptoms, but this is a high-risk procedure and results are variable.

Flashes and floaters

Flashes and floaters are very common symptoms, and in by far the majority of cases they are benign in origin and are due to posterior vitreous detachment. However, in some cases they can indicate retinal hole formation, which unchecked may lead to retinal detachment. The major causes of flashes and floaters are:

- Posterior vitreous detachment (PVD) ± retinal hole formation
- Vitreous haemorrhage
- Ocular migraine
- Posterior uveitis.

The flow chart in Figure 9.1 can be used to help to identify the cause of flashes and floaters.

Figure 9.1 Identifying the causes of flashes and floaters.

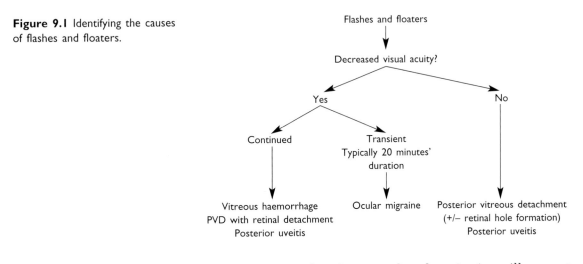

Posterior vitreous detachment and ocular migraine will account for over 90 per cent of the cases. The major concern for GPs seeing patients who experience flashes and floaters should be the possibility of retinal hole formation and the subsequent threat of retinal detachment. It is important to understand the relationship between the symptom complex of flashes and floaters, retinal hole formation and retinal detachment.

BASIC REFERRAL GUIDELINES

Retinal holes and small detachments are difficult to see with an ophthalmoscope, and referral is usually based on the history and symptoms alone. The most predictive indicator of serious pathology is associated permanent reduction in vision. A history of less than 6 weeks' duration is also important, but most of these patients will have only experienced a harmless posterior vitreous detachment without any sequelae.

- With long-standing floaters/flashes, there is no need for referral
- With floaters/flashes of less than 6 weeks' duration (especially in patients younger than 55 years of age, as this group of patients is too young to be affected by posterior vitreous detachment), an urgent outpatient referral is necessary
- If the floaters/flashes are of recent onset with decreased vision, an urgent eye casualty referral is vital.

POSTERIOR VITREOUS DETACHMENT

Action

Referral according to the guidelines above will allow diagnosis of the few cases that have an associated retinal hole or retinal detachment.

By far the most common cause of flashes and floaters, posterior vitreous detachment occurs in 75 per cent of the population over the age of 55 years, with perhaps 30 per cent being symptomatic. The vitreous body is a gel that fills the hollow posterior cavity of the eye behind the lens. It serves no particular function, and with increasing age it liquifies ('syneresis'). Eventually it collapses, imploding into the centre of the posterior cavity and detaching itself from the retina (Figure 9.2). Condensations within the vitreous body now cast shadows onto the retina, and these are often perceived as cobwebs or spider-shaped floaters. Tugging on the retina caused by the vitreous becoming detached is perceived as flashes of light. These symptoms fade with time.

Retinal hole formation

Posterior vitreous detachment is the single most common event associated with retinal hole formation. The vitreous in some eyes, especially myopes, is abnormally adherent to the retina in certain areas. A hole in the retina can then result when the vitreous fully detaches and pulls a piece of adherent retina with it (Figure 9.3). Trauma to the eye, including eye operations, will also disturb the vitreous gel and can lead to retinal detachment.

Figure 9.2 Posterior vitreous detachment.

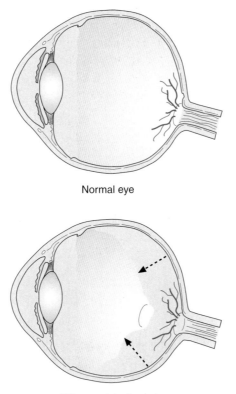

Normal eye

Vitreous detachment

Figure 9.3 Arrow-shaped retinal hole. Vitreous traction pulls open a tear, like pulling an old-style ring pull on a beer can.

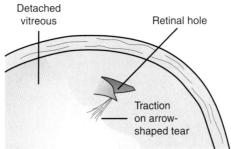

Detached
vitreous

Retinal hole

Traction
on arrow-
shaped tear

Action

A retinal hole can be sealed in the early stages by applying laser therapy around the hole to cause scar formation. This prevents any liquid vitreous from seeping through the hole and causing a retinal detachment.

Retinal detachment

If a retinal hole remains untreated liquid vitreous eventually percolates through the hole, gradually stripping off the retina

Figure 9.4 Liquid vitreous enters the retinal hole and gradually strips off the retina.

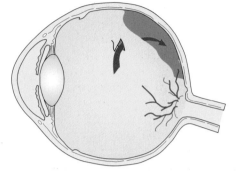

Figure 9.5 Retinal detachment crossing the macula. The advanced line of the detachment can be seen about to cross the fovea.

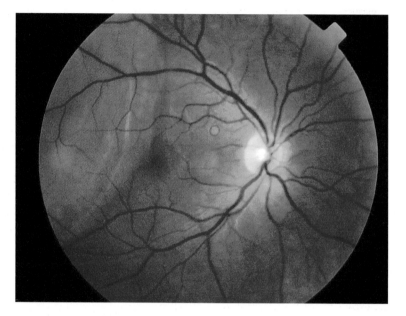

Action

Immediate referral to eye casualty department is indicated.

from the eye wall like peeling wallpaper (Figure 9.4). As more fluid flows through the hole the detachment creeps down from the periphery and will eventually cross the macula, with subsequent loss of central vision (Figure 9.5). During this stage patients may be aware of a dark curtain in the periphery of their vision. However, it is not uncommon for patients to fail to notice anything amiss until the detachment has crossed the macula and causes apparent sudden loss of vision. Surgery is then required to reattach the retina.

VITREOUS HAEMORRHAGE

Vitreous haemorrhage occurs when a retinal blood vessel bursts. This occurs in two specific situations:

<table>
<tr><td>

Findings

• Decreased visual acuity
• Loss of red reflex.

Action

Immediate referral to the eye casualty department is indicated. In patients where the view of the retina is obscured, periodic examination with ultrasound excludes the presence of a detachment. The haemorrhage usually clears spontaneously.

</td><td>

● As part of retinal hole formation; if the retinal tear cuts across a retinal blood vessel, a vitreous haemorrhage will be produced
● Rupture of new blood vessels, which form on the retina in conditions of ischaemia and are most often associated with proliferative diabetic retinopathy and as a complication of central retinal vein occlusion.

In both cases haemorrhage is perceived as a storm of floaters, which reduce visual acuity and, if a lot of blood is disgorged, may even cause a sudden loss of vision. Without a previous history of retinal vein thrombosis or proliferative diabetic retinopathy, the risk of retinal hole formation is very high.

OCULAR MIGRAINE

Classic symptoms of migraine such as headache and nausea are absent in some patients who complain of scintillating 'holes' in the vision or rhythmically flashing zigzag lines (Figure 9.6).

Attacks resolve spontaneously and typically last 20 minutes or so. It is important to realize that some patients have visual symptoms without any headache or nausea. No specific ophthalmological treatment is needed.

</td></tr>
</table>

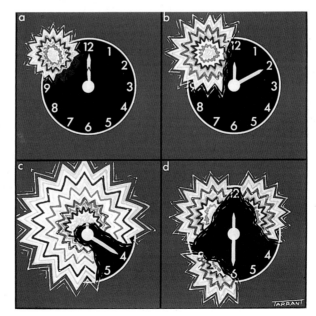

Figure 9.6 Artist's impression of an expanding migrainous scotoma. The lines would also be typically moving in a rhythmic fashion. Reproduced with permission from *Clinical Ophthalmology* by J. Kanski, 1999.

POSTERIOR UVEITIS

Action

Urgent referral is required for diagnosis and treatment of the primary pathology. Ocular inflammation is treated with corticosteriods injected around the eye.

Posterior uveitis is rare, and much less common than anterior uveitis. Patients are usually young adults, and complain of floaters. If associated macular oedema or dense vitreous inflammation occurs, vision will also be blurred.

On examination, opacities are evident in the vitreous and lesions on the retina may be seen, depending on the primary pathology. The most common causes are toxoplasmosis, sarcoidosis and pars planitis (see Glossary for details).

Double vision

Patients occasionally complain of double vision, but different patients mean different things when they say this, and the first job of the doctor is to define exactly what they do mean. Many patients merely mean blurred vision, while others genuinely mean seeing two of the same object. Once true double vision has been established, it is important to see if it is a binocular or monocular phenomenon. To ascertain this, the patient should shut one eye. If the double vision disappears, the symptom is clearly a binocular phenomenon.

The flow chart in Figure 10.1 can be used to help establish the cause of double vision.

Figure 10.1 Identifying the causes of double vision.

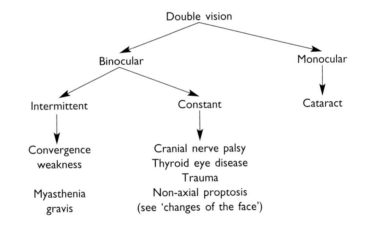

Action

All cases of double vision will need to be referred to the eye department. However, the diagnosis of painful third nerve palsy with a dilated pupil is an emergency requiring immediate referral to a neurosurgical unit. The cause is considered to be an intracranial aneurysm pressing on the third nerve until scanning has proven otherwise.

CONSTANT DOUBLE VISION

Cranial nerve palsy

There are three cranial nerves that control eye movements. Palsy of an individual nerve causes double vision, often with a characteristic appearance. Incomplete palsies are also common. These cause symptoms of double vision but may not be so obvious to clinical examination.

Third nerve palsy

Oculomotor (third) nerve palsy has a characteristic appearance (Figure 10.2):

● Divergent squint in primary position
● Variable amounts of ptosis
● The pupil may be normal, or it may be dilated and unreactive to light.

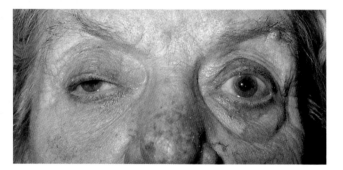

Figure 10.2 Third nerve palsy. Note the ptosis and divergent squint. It is essential to examine the pupil to determine whether it is dilated or not. Reproduced with permission from *Clinical Ophthalmology* by J. Kanski, 1999.

It is a relatively common condition in elderly people. The cause is usually vascular in nature, and is associated with diabetes and hypertension. The pupil is normal. Patients complain of sudden onset of double vision, which resolves spontaneously over the next 12 weeks or so. During this time, diplopia can be alleviated either by covering one eye with a patch or by incorporating temporary prisms into the patient's glasses.

More rarely, however, there is associated pain along with pupil dilatation. This indicates an aneurysm of the posterior communicating artery in the circle of Willis, pressing on the third nerve during its intracranial course (Figure 10.3). Patients with this condition are at high risk of subarachnoid haemorrhage, and require immediate investigation by a neurosurgeon. Only 30 per cent of patients survive if a subarachnoid haemorrhage occurs.

Figure 10.3 Aneurysm of the posterior communicating artery of the circle of Willis pressing on the third nerve. Reproduced with permission from *Clinical Ophthalmology* by J. Kanski, 1999.

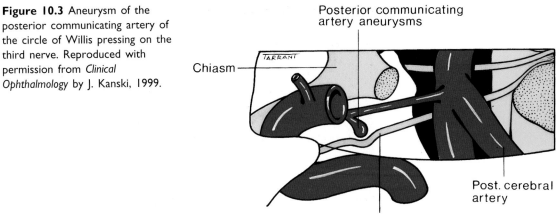

Sixth nerve palsy

Abducens (sixth) nerve palsy presents with sudden onset of diplopia associated with a convergent squint. Eye movements confirm paralysis of the lateral rectus muscle only. The cause is similar to that of third nerve palsies, although it is not associated with intracranial aneurysms. The condition will typically resolve spontaneously over 12–20 weeks.

Fourth nerve palsy

Patients with trochlear (fourth) nerve palsy complain of difficulty with reading or looking down, and occasionally of torsional diplopia (Figure 10.4). It usually occurs after some kind of trauma to the head. Eye movements usually appear normal, but occasionally underaction of the superior oblique muscle can be detected with the naked eye (Figure 10.5).

Figure 10.4 Torsional diplopia.

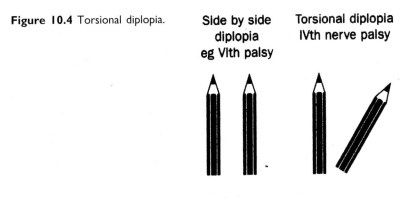

Trauma is the most common cause of trochlear nerve palsy, and it is therefore seen most often in young men. Again, spontaneous resolution is common, but some patients may require corrective surgery.

Figure 10.5 Right fourth nerve palsy. The right eye underacts on looking down and to the left. Reproduced with permission from *Clinical Ophthalmology* by J. Kanski, 1999.

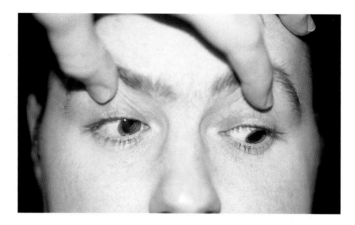

Thyroid eye disease

During the acute phase of thyroid eye disease, the extraocular muscles are infiltrated with lymphocytes and can swell to eight times their normal size (Figure 10.6). This bulk causes proptosis as well as restricting normal eye movements. Double vision is common, especially in up gaze.

Figure 10.6 CT scan showing enlarged extraocular muscles. The optic nerve can be squeezed and damaged at the apex of the orbit. Reproduced with permission from *Clinical Ophthalmology* by J. Kanski, 1999.

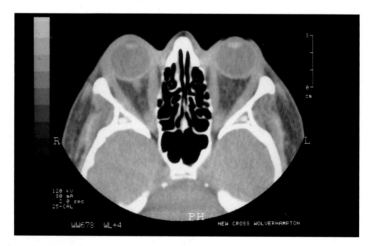

Action

The eye department should follow up all cases of thyroid eye disease with double vision or proptosis.

Later in the disease process, the lymphocytes are replaced with scar tissue. The unpredictable nature of this process can lead to bizarre positions of the eye and difficulties with double vision. During the active phase, radiotherapy, immunosuppression and orbital decompression are used to reduce muscle infiltration and double vision. During the 'burnt out' phase, i.e. when all the lymphocytes have been replaced with scar tissue, surgery is used to try to re-establish binocular single vision.

Trauma

Trauma in the vicinity of the cheekbone can cause fractures of the orbital floor (Figure 10.7). Initially there may be dramatic orbital haemorrhage and swelling of the eyelids, but once this subsides double vision may be become evident, especially on up gaze. The inferior rectus muscle becomes trapped in the fracture, preventing adequate up gaze (Figure 10.8).

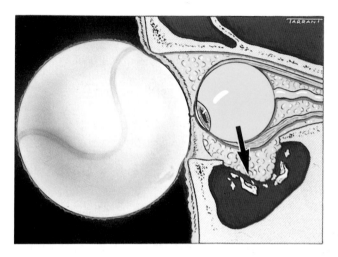

Figure 10.7 Blow-out fracture of the orbit. Reproduced with permission from *Clinical Ophthalmology* by J. Kanski, 1999.

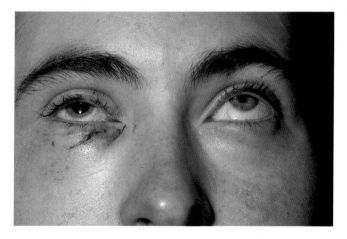

Figure 10.8 Poor upgaze after blow-out fracture. Reproduced with permission from *Clinical Ophthalmology* by J. Kanski, 1999.

> *Action*
>
> Surgery within the first 2 weeks has the best chance of releasing trapped tissue and restoring single vision.

INTERMITTENT DOUBLE VISION

Convergence weakness

Some patients, usually young, complain of blurring of vision or frank diplopia on reading. Orthoptic testing shows their eye convergence to be poor. Treatment relies on eye exercises.

Myasthenia gravis

This is a rare autoimmune condition that frequently affects the eyes, typically in the third and fourth decades. The cardinal symptoms are intermittent double vision and variable ptosis of the lids. The muscles controlling both movements are easily fatigued.

Action

Although patients may present to an ophthalmology department for assessment of double vision, it is likely that a neurologist will handle their case. Various drug treatments can be helpful in alleviating symptoms, and some patients require thymectomy.

Part II

Change in appearance

Introduction to change in appearance

The predominant feature in the history is quite often a change from the patient's normal appearance. In many cases of change in appearance, the diagnosis is simply a matter of pattern recognition. The conditions have been divided anatomically as well as by mode of presentation:

- Changes of the face
    - Acutely inflamed
        Herpes zoster ophthalmicus
        Orbital cellulitis
        Dacryocystitis
        Acutely prominent eyes (proptosis)
    - Uninflamed
        Facial palsy
        Prominent eyes (proptosis)
- Changes of the eyelids
    Acutely inflamed (meibomium cyst, stye, drug-induced dermatitis)
    Uninflamed (ptosis, lumps and bumps)
- Changes of the conjunctiva
    Acutely inflamed (see Chapter 16)
    Uninflamed (pterygium, lipodermoid, conjunctival retention cyst, pigmented lesions)
- Changes of the pupil and iris
    One pupil bigger than the other
    Changes of the iris.

Changes of the face

ACUTELY INFLAMED

Herpes zoster ophthalmicus

Most doctors will be familiar with the typical appearance of herpes zoster ophthalmicus (shingles; Figure 12.1). Involvement of the eye occurs in about 50 per cent of cases, and is particularly associated with herpes lesions on the side of the nose ('Hutchinson sign'). This demonstrates involvement of the nasociliary branch of the trigeminal nerve. Eye complications vary from conjunctivitis to uveitis and keratitis. Uveitis occurs in about 40 per cent of cases, and correct treatment prevents further complications.

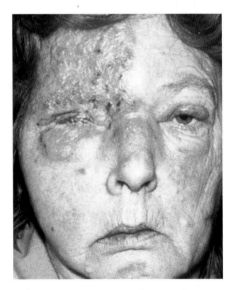

Figure 12.1 Herpes zoster ophthalmicus (shingles).

> *Action*
>
> Systemic treatment with famciclovir 250 mg three times daily for 1 week
>   Topical acyclovir and fusidin-H (hydrocortisone 1%, fusidic acid 2%) three times daily until the crusts have separated
>   Referral to the eye department within 1 week to check for ocular complications.

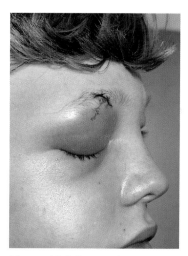

Figure 12.2 Preseptal cellulitis. There is no proptosis, and if the lid is opened eye movements are found to be normal. Reproduced with permission from *Clinical Ophthalmology* by J. Kanski, 1999.

Figure 12.3 Orbital cellulitis. Most cases occur in children and young adults, and are frequently related to sinus disease. However, infection post-orbital trauma, including operations, is occasionally the cause. Reproduced with permission from *Clinical Ophthalmology* by J. Kanski, 1999.

Preseptal cellulitis

Preseptal cellulitis is a subcutaneous infection that is superficial to the orbital septum and it is generally caused by an infected local laceration or insect bite (Figure 10.2). Spread of oedema from local infections such as herpes zoster ophthalmicus (HZO) or dacryocystitis is another common cause (see Figure 12.1).

> **Action**
>
> The patient is febrile and requires treatment with oral penicillin.

Orbital cellulitis

In contrast, orbital cellulitis is an infection of the soft tissues behind the orbital septum. The resulting oedema restricts eye movements and causes a painful proptosis (Figure 12.3).

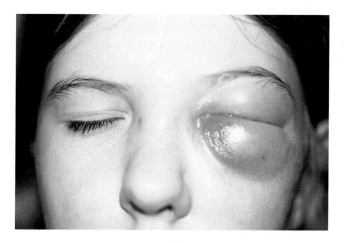

> **Action**
>
> Patients do not look well and they need hospital admission for intravenous antibiotics and evaluation for potential abscess drainage.

Dacryocystitis

This is caused by infection of the lacrimal sac secondary to obstruction of the nasolacrimal duct. The clinical picture of a tender abscess on the side of the nose just below the medial end of the eye is classic (see Chapter 19). Watering of the eye will occur, and will continue until an operation reinstates drainage of tears.

Action

Systemic broad-spectrum antibiotics and warm compresses should be prescribed. Referral to an ophthalmologist is required for definitive surgery in the form of a dacryocystrhinostomy (DCR). This operation establishes a new connection between the sac and the nose, once again allowing the free flow of tears.

Acutely prominent eyes (proptosis)

The commonest cause of both bilateral and unilateral proptosis is thyroid eye disease, and in some cases the eyes can appear quite inflamed (Figure 12.4). Other causes include orbital cellulitis (see above), inflammations of other orbital structures such as the lacrimal gland, and carotid–cavernous fistula. Because the orbit is distended, eye movements are usually restricted.

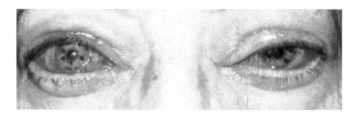

Figure 12.4 Thyroid eye disease. The eyes are proptotic and inflamed, with lid oedema.

Action

All cases require urgent referral for accurate diagnosis and appropriate treatment. In extreme cases, compression of the optic nerve can threaten visual function (see Chapter 21).

UNINFLAMED

Facial palsy

Seventh nerve palsy (Bell's palsy) is usually idiopathic, but can be secondary to tumours such as cholesteotoma and acoustic neuroma. With this in mind, patients whose seventh

Figure 12.5 Facial palsy. Despite attempted closure, the left eye remains unprotected.

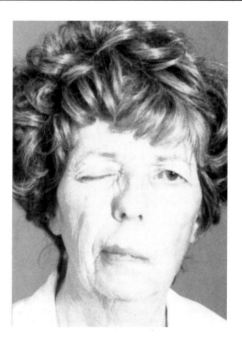

Action

Initial treatment should focus on protecting the cornea, and includes prescribing copious artificial tears and taping the eye shut at night. A temporary tarsorrophy may be required to prevent exposure (Figure 12.6). If simple measures fail to keep the eye comfortable, urgent referral to the eye department is justified. Long term, once the degree of recovery has been established, further surgery to improve both cosmesis and function is usually possible.

nerve palsy shows no sign of resolution should be referred to an ENT specialist. Problems with the eye can develop because of poor eye closure (Figure 12.5). Exposure-type corneal ulcers can develop, causing a great deal of discomfort. The cornea has three defence mechanisms:

- Lid closure and blink reflex (controlled by the seventh nerve)
- Reflex watering (controlled by the seventh nerve)
- Corneal sensation, which triggers both of the above (controlled by the fifth nerve).

If two of these mechanisms are out of action problems are likely to develop, and this is quite common, as the seventh nerve controls two mechanisms. Loss of corneal sensation is usually disastrous.

Figure 12.6 Temporary tarsorrophy. The eyelids are stitched together to reduce exposure.

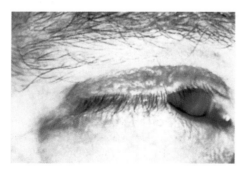

Prominent eyes (proptosis)

Without associated inflammation, patients do not always appreciate prominence of the eyes. Unilateral proptosis, however, is usually more obvious. The commonest cause of both unilateral and bilateral proptosis is thyroid eye disease. Tumours within the muscle cone will push the eye directly forward ('axial proptosis'), while those outside the cone will displace the globe in any direction, commonly causing double vision (Figure 12.7). Proptosis should always be taken seriously and deserves further investigation and possibly CT or MRI scanning.

Figure 12.7 Proptosis with displacement of the globe inferiorly. The patient complained of double vision, and scanning revealed a frontal sinus mucocele. Reproduced with permission from *Clinical Ophthalmology* by J. Kanski, 1999.

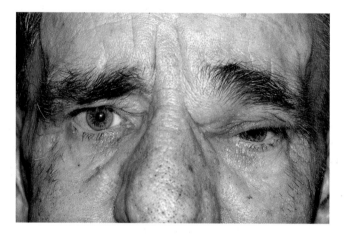

There are many possible causes:

- Thyroid eye disease
- Tumours arising from tissues within the orbit
    Vascular malformations
    Meningioma/gliomas (nerves)
    Rhabdomyosarcoma (muscle)
- Sinus mucoceles
- Dermoid cyst.

Changes of the eyelids

ACUTELY INFLAMED

Meibomium cyst (tarsal cyst/chalazion)

This is an abscess in the lid caused by infection of stagnated sebaceous secretions secondary to blockage of the meibomium gland orifice (Figure 13.1). Patients with acne rosacea and seborrhoeic dermatitis are at increased risk of cyst formation. Once the infection fades, a non-tender hard lump may remain (chalazion).

Figure 13.1 Inflamed meibomium cyst. Patients present to the doctor with a tender lump in the eyelid 1–2 mm away from the lash line.

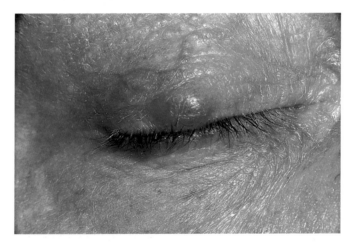

Action

In most cases the infection settles itself, but using hot compresses to encourage the meibomium orifices to open and release infected material can speed up this process. Persistent lumps can be referred for surgical removal (Figure 13.2). In atypical cases the excised material should be sent for pathological examination as, very rarely, sebaceous cell carcinoma can masquerade as a tarsal cyst.

Figure 13.2 Incision and drainage of a cyst. In young patients who will not tolerate excision under local anaesthesia, persistent lumps should be simply observed unless they are very bad. In most cases the lump will eventually resolve, perhaps over 6–8 months. Reproduced with permission from *Clinical Ophthalmology* by J. Kanski, 1999.

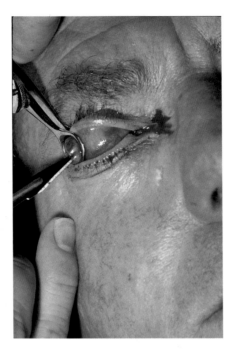

Stye

This is an infection of the lash root and is often associated with a mild preseptal cellulitis (Figure 13.3).

Figure 13.3 Stye. There is a tender swelling of the lid, with abscess formation at the lash root. Reproduced with permission from *Clinical Ophthalmology* by J. Kanski, 1999.

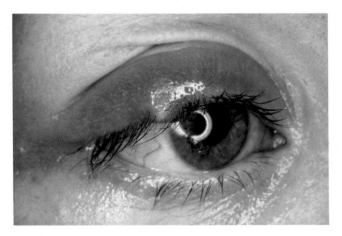

Action

No treatment is required in most cases, but epilation of the associated lash and hot compresses will encourage drainage of pus.

Figure 13.4 Allergic dermatitis. The main offenders are chloramphenicol and neomycin. Neomycin is contained in the preparation Betnesol-N, which is frequently used in the UK following cataract surgery.

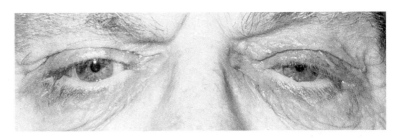

Drug-induced allergic dermatitis

This is a common, usually bilateral, condition frequently caused by sensitivity to eye drops (Figure 13.4).

> **Action**
>
> Removal of the offending eye drops will solve the problem.

UNINFLAMED

Droopy lids (Ptosis)

This is a common complaint amongst older patients, which can also occasionally follow intraocular surgery. By far and away the majority are due to stretching of the upper lid levator muscle tendon ('aponeurosis defect'). One or both upper lids may droop to obscure a view of the upper iris, and may even obscure a view of the pupil (Figure 13.5). In an effort to keep

Figure 13.5 Unilateral ptosis of the right eye. Reproduced with permission from *Clinical Ophthalmology* by J. Kanski, 1999.

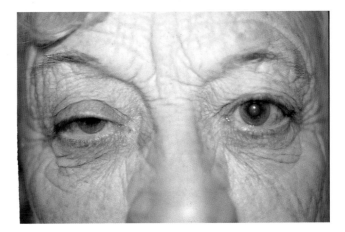

the upper lids raised sufficiently, frontalis muscle overaction is commonly seen, causing a raised eyebrow and lines across the forehead. Excess skin hanging over the upper lids ('dermatochalasis') can cause a pseudoptosis (Figure 13.6). Other causes of ptosis are relatively rare, and include:

- Neurogenic
    Third nerve palsy – associated divergent squint and double vision
    Horner syndrome – associated ipsilateral small pupil
- Myogenic
    Myasthenia gravis – associated with variable lid position and frequently with double vision.

Figure 13.6 Dermatochalasis causing pseudoptosis. Reproduced with permission from *Clinical Ophthalmology* by J. Kanski, 1999.

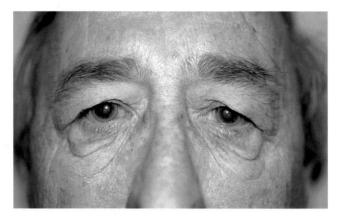

Action

If the drooping upper lid starts to obscure vision or looks unsightly, then surgical correction is possible. Excessive dermatochalasis is simply treated by excision of excess skin.

Lumps and bumps

These are generally recognized by their typical appearance. Most require excision for cosmetic reasons only, while a few are removed because of a suspicion of malignancy. They include:

- Papilloma (Figure 13.7)
- Xanthelasma (Figure 13.8)
- Cyst of Moll (Figure 13.9)
- Cyst of Zeis (Figure 13.10)
- Milia (Figure 13.11)

Figure 13.7 Papilloma. This is common and has a distinctive appearance. Reproduced with permission from *Clinical Ophthalmology* by J. Kanski, 1999.

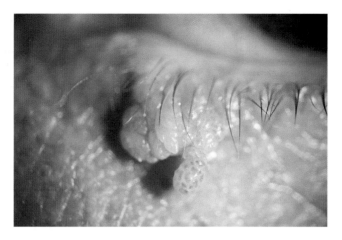

Figure 13.8 Xanthelasma. This may occasionally indicate hypercholesterolaemia. Reproduced with permission from *Clinical Ophthalmology* by J. Kanski, 1999.

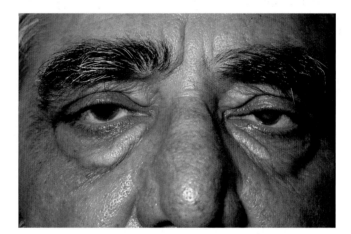

Figure 13.9 Cyst of Moll. These are common lesions on the lid margin with a small, round, translucent appearance. They are fluid filled, and a simple stab with a needle is usually all that is required. The larger lesion in this photograph is also a fluid-filled cyst, but is derived from 'normal skin' as opposed to eyelid structures and represents a sweat gland hydrocystoma. Reproduced with permission from *Clinical Ophthalmology* by J. Kanski, 1999.

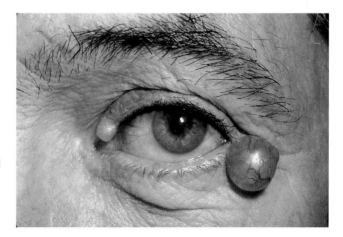

Figure 13.10 Cyst of Zeis. This is similar to a cyst of Moll but is not translucent, as it is filled with oily secretions. Reproduced with permission from *Clinical Ophthalmology* by J. Kanski, 1999.

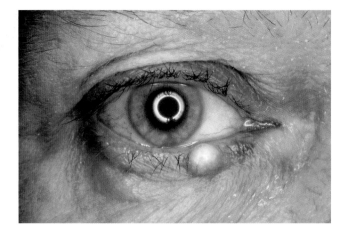

Figure 13.11 Milia, which are crops of tiny white cysts. Reproduced with permission from *Clinical Ophthalmology* by J. Kanski, 1999.

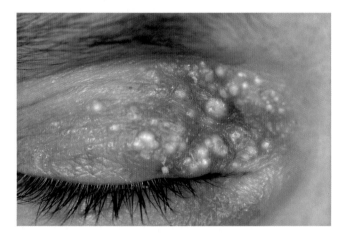

Figure 13.12 Keratoacanthoma. Reproduced with permission from *Clinical Ophthalmology* by J. Kanski, 1999.

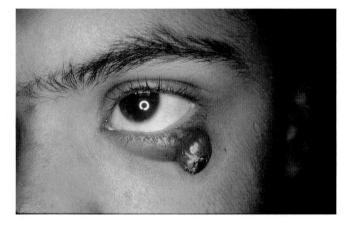

- Cutaneous horn (Figure 13.15)
- Keratocanthoma (Figure 13.12)
- Basal cell carcinoma (Figure 13.13)
- Squamous cell carcinoma.

Keratoacanthoma

Keratoacanthomas are relatively uncommon, but deserve mention as they cause otherwise healthy patients a great deal of distress over the often unspoken fear of malignancy (Figure 13.12). This reputation is achieved by way of its rapid growth – it can double in size over a few days. Simple excision is all that is required.

Basal cell carcinoma (rodent ulcer)

Basal cell carcinoma (BCC) is the most common human malignancy, and accounts for 90 per cent of all eyelid tumours. The condition generally affects the elderly, although younger patients in their thirties and forties with fair skin and high levels of sun exposure are increasingly affected. The lower lid is the commonest site. The tumours are slow growing and non-metastasizing. However, left untreated they will ulcerate and eat away (hence 'rodent') a large portion of the eyelid (Figure 13.13). The typical signs of the tumour are (Figure 13.14):

- A raised pearly lesion
- Central ulceration
- Raised rolled edges
- Dilated blood vessels coursing over the tumour
- Loss of eyelashes.

Figure 13.13 Extensive rodent ulcer involving most of the lower lid. If untreated, these will eventually erode into the orbit and neighbouring sinuses. Reproduced with permission from *Clinical Ophthalmology* by J. Kanski, 1999.

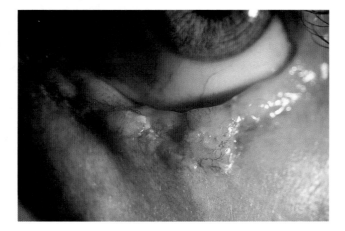

Figure 13.14 Basal cell carcinoma. Note the ulcerated centre and loss of eyelashes. Reproduced with permission from *Clinical Ophthalmology* by J. Kanski, 1999.

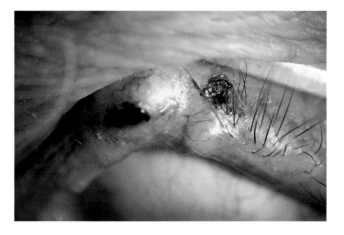

> **Action**
>
> Early referral is indicated for complete excision. Large portions of the lids are frequently sacrificed to achieve complete excision, and these require complicated oculoplastic reconstruction of the eyelid defects.

Squamous cell carcinoma

Often clinically indistinguishable from BCCs, these are usually diagnosed by the pathologist. Occasionally they present as a cutaneous horn (Figure 13.15). Metastasis to the lymph nodes can occur, so complete tumour excision is necessary.

Figure 13.15 Cutaneous horn. Some are merely associated actinic keratosis. Reproduced with permission from *Clinical Ophthalmology* by J. Kanski, 1999.

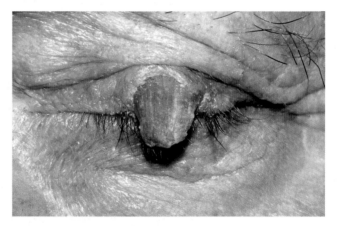

Changes of the conjunctiva

INFLAMED

See Chapter 16.

UNINFLAMED

All the conditions below have typical appearances, and any atypical lesions observed should be referred for further assessment.

Pterygium

Action

In cosmetically bad cases these lesions can be removed; however, there is a propensity for recurrence. There is no malignant potential.

Literally meaning 'wing-like', pterygium is a triangular growth of conjunctiva over the surface of the cornea (Figure 14.1). It is related to sun damage and is commonest in hot climates, but none the less does occur in the UK. Patients complain of an unsightly appearance or sometimes of continual redness of the conjunctiva. A similar lesion that does not encroach onto the cornea is called a pinguecula (Figure 14.2).

Figure 14.1 Advanced pterygium. Reproduced with permission from *Clinical Ophthalmology* by J. Kanski, 1999.

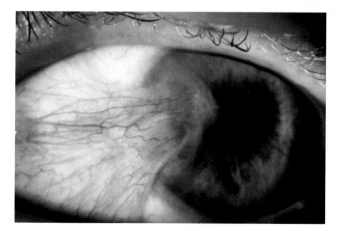

Figure 14.2 Pinguecula.
Reproduced with permission from
Clinical Ophthalmology by J. Kanski,
1999.

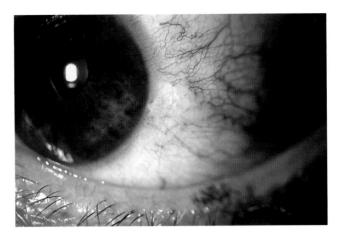

Lipodermoid (dermolipoma)

Lipodermoids present in adult life as soft conjunctival masses located in the lateral canthal area (Figure 14.3).

Figure 14.3 Lipodermoid. The patient has to look in the opposite direction for the lesion to be observed. Reproduced with permission from *Clinical Ophthalmology* by J. Kanski, 1999.

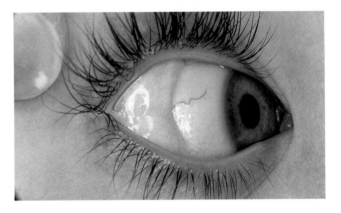

Action

Lipodermoids are benign but should not be removed, as postoperative scarring will cause difficulties with ocular motility. If the lesion is salmon pink-coloured referral is indicated, as this is an indication of conjunctival lymphoma.

Action

If large, treatment is effected by simple puncture of the cyst wall with a needle.

Conjunctival retention cyst

Conjunctival retention cysts are very common and are generally asymptomatic thin-walled lesions containing fluid (Figure 14.4).

Figure 14.4 Conjunctival
retention cyst. Reproduced with
permission from *Clinical
Ophthalmology* by J. Kanski, 1999.

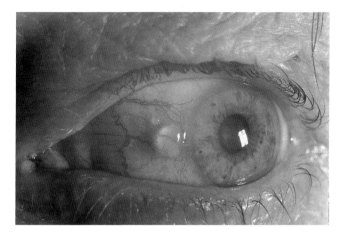

Pigmented lesions

A pigmented lesion always raises concern because of the
possibility of melanoma. However, conjunctival melanoma is
very rare below the age of 50 years, and is also very rare in
dark-skinned races. The causes of pigmentation are:

● Naevi
● Epithelial (racial) melanosis
● Melanoma.

Conjunctival naevi

This is a benign unilateral condition that presents in the first
two decades of life. Lesions can be slightly elevated and
contain variable amounts of pigment. Typical locations are
next to the corneal limbus (Figure 14.5) or on the caruncle.

Figure 14.5 Conjunctival naevus
at the corneal limbus. Small round
cystic areas within the naevus are
typical and reassuring. Reproduced
with permission from *Clinical
Ophthalmology* by J. Kanski, 1999.

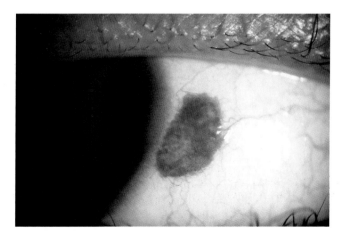

Growth may occur during puberty, but after this it is a sign of malignant transformation.

> **Action**
>
> Many patients request removal of these lesions for cosmetic reasons, and this is simply done.

Conjunctival epithelial (racial) melanosis

> **Action**
>
> Reassurance is all that is required.

This is an entirely benign bilateral, although asymmetrical, condition that is frequently present amongst blacks and other individuals with a dark complexion. Presentation is during the first few years of life and is stable by adulthood.

Conjunctival melanoma

This is a rare tumour presenting in the sixth decade with a pigmented nodule fixed to the sclera (Figure 14.6).

Figure 14.6 Conjunctival melanoma. Reproduced with permission from *Clinical Ophthalmology* by J. Kanski, 1999.

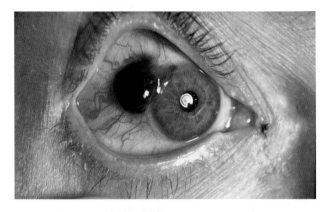

> **Action**
>
> Urgent referral for excision is necessary.

Changes of the pupil and iris

ONE PUPIL IS BIGGER THAN THE OTHER

A difference in size between the pupils can occasionally cause alarm amongst patients. In by far the majority of cases the cause is Adie pupil, which is benign.

Although this is the common presentation, pupil sizes are relative to one another and the first task is to decide which pupil is abnormal – the big one or the little one.

- Adie pupil is an abnormally large pupil
- Previous trauma may cause an abnormally large pupil
- Horner's syndrome is an abnormally small pupil with an associated ptosis
- Argyll Robertson pupil is an abnormally small pupil.

Horner's syndrome is rare, and consists of a small pupil associated with a 2-mm ptosis on the same side (Figure 15.1). If this is suspected, patients should be referred for further examination and elucidation of the primary cause, of which there are many. Argyll Robertson pupil is mentioned in most medical textbooks and is caused by neurosyphilis. However, it is so rare in the UK that neither the author nor anyone else he knows has seen a case!

Figure 15.1 Right Horner's syndrome. Reproduced with permission from *Clinical Ophthalmology* by J. Kanski, 1999.

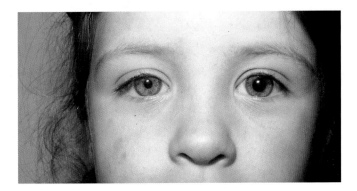

Adie pupil

This is quite common, and generally affects young adult females. The cause is denervation of the pupillary muscle, and it is probably of viral aetiology. The features are:

- A large, regular pupil
- A poor or absent direct light reflex
- Diminished tendon reflexes (Holmes Adie syndrome).

Previous trauma

Direct trauma to the eye (for instance a squash ball injury) can cause rupture of the pupillary muscle, leading to a dilated and poorly reacting pupil.

It is important to realize that a dilated pupil is not a sign of raised intracranial pressure or tumour in a fully conscious patient.

CHANGES OF THE IRIS

Various pigmented and non-pigmented tumours of the iris occur, but they are rather rare. Iris naevi are very common, but are generally flat and less than 3 mm in size. Melanomas of the iris are very slow growing, with low malignant potential. Distortion of the pupil margin is a sign of malignancy (Figue 15.2).

Figure 15.2 Iris melanoma distorting the pupil margin. Reproduced with permission from *Clinical Ophthalmology* by J. Kanski, 1999.

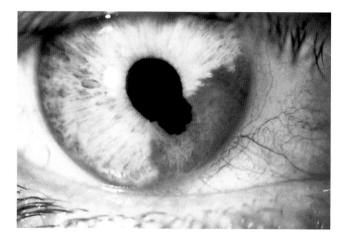

Part III

Red/painful/irritable eyes

Red and painful eyes

These two complaints have been grouped together for the simple reason that they often present together. In some circumstances they do appear in isolation, and that is why they have been subdivided into separate sections of this chapter. However, it is important to realize their inter-relationship, and that patients do not always complain about the same condition in the same way. For instance, while one patient with acute glaucoma may complain of an acutely red eye that is painful, another may simply complain of a very painful eye and leave the observation of redness to the doctor. The point here is that, in establishing the diagnosis of the acute red and/or painful eye, all the conditions in both sections need to be considered in case the patient muddies the waters with an atypical history.

While the majority of conditions seen in the primary care setting with these symptoms will be trivial, some causes are very serious and threaten the long-term function of the eye – vision. These include:

- Acute glaucoma
- Corneal ulcer
- Dendritic ulcer
- Endophthalmitis.

One of the main aims of this chapter is to arm the primary care physician with the key points in the history and examination that will allow confident diagnosis and referral of these conditions.

THE RED EYE

The common causes of a red eye in primary care are:

- Conjunctivitis
  Bacterial
  Viral
  Chlamydial
- Episcleritis

- Subconjunctival haemorrhage
- Iritis.

Rarer causes of red eye are:

- Acute glaucoma
- Corneal ulcer
- Dendritic ulcer
- Scleritis
- Endophthalmitis.

History

Three important features in the history can help to narrow the diagnosis:

- Laterality (see Figure 16.1)
- Stickiness
- Pain.

It is also important to ask about any ophthalmic history, and in particular about any recent eye operations such as cataract surgery. Endophthalmitis is a very rare complication of intraocular surgery (see complications of cataract surgery in Chapter 7) that presents as an increasingly red and painful eye post-surgery. Visual acuity is also markedly reduced.

Figure 16.1 Identifying the causes of red and painful eyes.

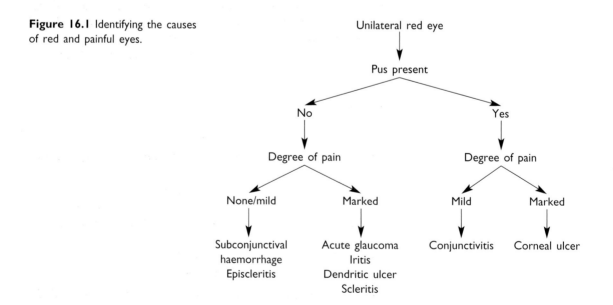

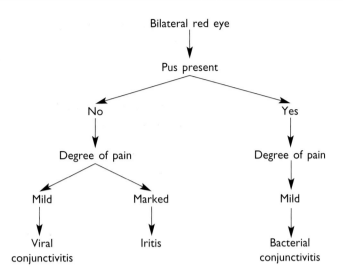

Note that serious causes of the red eye all present with marked pain and affect only one eye.

The location of the pain is helpful. Pain caused by high intraocular pressure (acute glaucoma) is universally referred to the eyebrow and not the eye. To establish this, ask the patient where the pain is and if there is acute glaucoma he or she will dutifully point to the eyebrow. If not, the patient will tell you that the pain is in or on the eye.

It is important to question the patient closely to find out if pus has been present. If both eyes are red and there is pus, the diagnosis is almost certainly conjunctivitis. Corneal ulcers are almost invariably unilateral, and can be distinguished from unilateral conjunctivitis – which is more common than often assumed – by examination of the cornea (see below)

Examination

The examination should focus on the:

- Visual acuity – if significantly reduced, it suggests corneal damage
- Eyelids – presence of mucopus can be confirmed
- Conjunctiva – search for follicles in the inferior fornix
- Corneal sensation – if markedly decreased, this suggests a dendritic ulcer
- Cornea – to exclude corneal ulcers
- Pupil – to exclude acute glaucoma.

If the visual acuity, cornea and pupil are normal, none of the four serious eye conditions is present.

The easiest of the three serious causes to exclude is acute glaucoma. This is because 100 per cent of cases will have an abnormal pupil, which is easily spotted if looked for (see below). During an attack of acute glaucoma, the pupil is always mid-dilated and does not react to light.

Bacterial corneal ulceration is usually obvious to gross inspection of the cornea, although a magnifying glass and fluorescein staining will aid in the diagnosis. Dendritic ulceration is often more subtle, especially in early and therefore small ulcers. Both magnification and fluorescein staining will often be required.

As a rule of thumb, an eye with decreasing vision or pain that is worsening each day should be referred to an eye casualty unit.

RED EYE WITH PUS

Conjunctivitis

Conjunctivitis associated with pus has two main causes: acute bacterial infection or chlamydial infection. Primary viral conjunctivitis may become secondarily infected with bacteria.

Bacterial conjunctivitis

Acute bacterial conjunctivitis is common, and can be bilateral or unilateral. Typically there is a mucopurulent discharge causing stickiness and gluey eyelids in the morning. Patients may describe the eye as feeling gritty or hot with variable amounts of watering.

Mucopus is evident on the lids. Once all the mucopus has been removed, vision is not affected. The cornea and pupil are normal.

Findings

- Mucopus is evident on the lids
- The cornea is normal.

Action

The condition is self-limiting, resolving within 1–2 weeks, and antibiotic drops merely hasten this process – this is important to understand in cases of conjunctivitis that do not readily resolve. Topical chloramphenicol every 2 hours supplemented with chloramphenicol ointment at night is effective in most cases. Treatment should last at least 5 days, and may be tapered to four times a day once the initial infection is controlled.

Conjunctivitis that does not improve after 2 weeks

First check that an important diagnosis has not been missed and exclude other causes of conjunctivitis, e.g. chlamydia and viruses, including molluscum contagiosum. Worrying features in the history are a unilateral red eye, increasing pain, decreased vision and the absence of pus.

- Check the diagnosis
- Ensure that the patient has complied with treatment
- Resist the temptation to prescribe a different antibiotic – resistance to broad-spectrum antibiotic drops is extremely rare
- Stop treatment or refer, rather than prescribe a different antibiotic. Drug toxicity is a common sustaining feature in chronic cases of conjunctivitis (see Chapter 17)
- Treat any associated blepharitis (see Chapter 17).

Because conjunctivitis is self-limiting, cessation of all treatment may be all that is required.

Molluscum contagiosum

This viral infection is most common in children and manifests as crops of nodules, usually on the trunk. In adults it is a rare cause of chronic conjunctivitis.

Findings

- Follicles in the conjunctiva
- A pale waxy nodule close to eye is typical (Figure 16.2).

Action

Resolution is rapid with cautery or excision of the nodule.

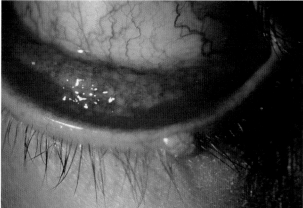

Figure 16.2 Molluscum contagiosum. Note the lesion on the eyelid margin and the follicular (tapioca pudding appearance) reaction in the lower conjunctival sac. Reproduced with permission from *Clinical Ophthalmology* by J. Kanski, 1999.

<table>
<tr><td>

Findings

The clinical picture is similar to acute bilateral conjunctivitis; however, chlamydial conjunctivitis is distinguished by:
- Large follicles in the inferior conjunctiva
- Preauricular lymphadenopathy.

</td></tr>
</table>

Chlamydial conjunctivitis

Typically this affects young adults during their sexually active years, but is far less common than bacterial conjunctivitis. The infection is almost invariably venereal, with conjunctivitis occurring 1 week after sexual contact. There may be associated urethritis or cervicitis.

> **Action**
>
> Systemic treatment is needed with oral tetracycline such as oxytetracycline 100 mg daily for 1–2 weeks. Patients should be referred to a sexually transmitted diseases clinic for contact tracing, otherwise re-infection may occur.

<table>
<tr><td>

Findings

- The cornea is abnormal, with a yellowish-white opaque area (Figure 16.3)
- There is a mucopurulent discharge, often with a hypopyon (Figure 16.4).

</td></tr>
</table>

Bacterial corneal ulcer

Any damage to the corneal epithelium, for example after trauma, has the potential to become an infected ulcer. Wearing contact lenses increases the risk of corneal ulceration. Infected ulcers are more common among elderly and infirm individuals, in whom presentation may be delayed. The eye is markedly painful and red as well as being sticky.

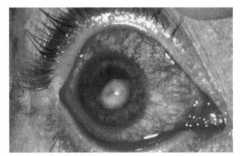

Figure 16.3 Bacterial corneal ulcer.

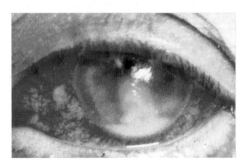

Figure 16.4 Hypopyon. This is a precipitate of inflammatory cells causing a fluid level in the inferior anterior chamber, and its presence signals severe, active intraocular inflammation.

Action

These ulcers are sight threatening, and require immediate referral. Once in hospital, scrapes from the ulcer are taken for culture and antibiotic sensitivities while the patient is put on intensive antibiotic drop therapy. Fortified gentamicin and cefuroxime are often chosen, as they are effective against most gram positive and negative bacteria. The infection affects the deeper layers of the cornea, and so healing will lead to a degree of scarring often associated with in growth of blood vessels into the cornea. Both of these processes can interrupt the clear visual pathway and so cause permanent visual loss.

RED EYE WITHOUT PUS

If there is a red eye with no history of mucopurulent discharge, the threshold for referral should be lowered and conditions such as iritis, dendritic ulcer and acute glaucoma considered. Marked pain increases the likelihood of these conditions.

Iritis (anterior uveitis)

Iritis is an intraocular inflammation affecting the iris and ciliary body, and presents as a unilateral painful red eye often associated with photophobia (bilateral cases are very rare). There is never a history of stickiness. Without the correct diagnosis and treatment, the pain increases daily. After 5–6 days patients usually present spontaneously to eye casualty, often with a story of failed treatment for conjunctivitis. If there is a protracted delay in diagnosis, posterior synechiae may form. These are areas where the pupil becomes stuck to the

Figure 16.5 'Cloverleaf' pupil caused by dilating the pupil in the presence of posterior synechiae. Reproduced with permission from *Clinical Ophthalmology* by J. Kanski, 1999.

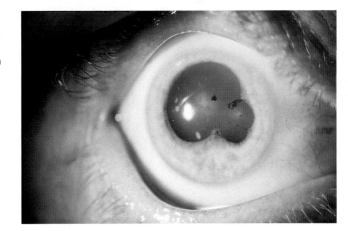

Findings
• There is no mucopus
• The pupil is in spasm in uveitis and therefore constricted
• Iris details may be slightly blurred compared with the other eye due to inflammatory debris in the anterior chamber
• When the inflammation is severe, clumps of inflammatory cells (keratic precipitates) may be seen adhering to the back of the cornea (Figure 16.6). Magnification is usually required to see them.

lens, and this will give a cloverleaf pattern to the iris when it is dilated (Figure 16.5).

Iritis is a recurrent condition, and patients second time around usually know what the diagnosis is.

Much is made in undergraduate textbooks of circumciliary injection and presence of posterior synechiae. However, the former is an unreliable sign of uveitis, and the latter will only be seen after dilating the pupil.

Action
Patients should be referred to the eye department immediately for intensive treatment with topical corticosteroid drops. These should not be prescribed in the primary care setting unless a diagnosis of dendritic ulcer can be confidently excluded (see below). Most cases respond rapidly to treatment and settle fully after 4–6 weeks of treatment. In a minority of cases the inflammatory process grumbles on despite treatment, in which case the patient may have to use corticosteroid drops on a permanent basis. Most cases of anterior uveitis are idiopathic, but occasionally the condition is a sign of systemic disease – most notably ankylosing spondylitis and sarcoidosis.

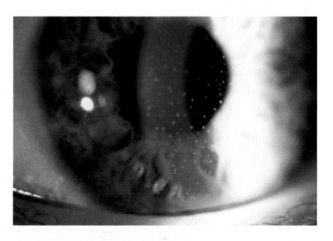

Figure 16.6 Keratic precipitates stuck to the inside of the cornea. In severe attacks, a hypopyon may form. Reproduced with permission from *Clinical Ophthalmology* by J. Kanski, 1999.

Dendritic ulcer

Dendritic ulcer (from the Greek *dendron*: tree) is a herpes simplex infection of the cornea. It is analogous to a cold sore – it represents the reactivation of latent virus from the trigeminal ganglion, but in a rather more devastating location. As with bacterial ulcers the deeper layers of the cornea can be affected, especially after recurrent attacks, and so even with

Figure 16.7 Corneal scarring with vascularization of the cornea. Reproduced with permission from *Clinical Ophthalmology* by J. Kanski, 1999.

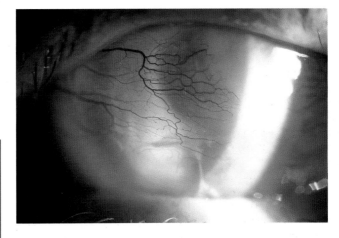

Findings

- There is no mucopus
- Corneal sensation is markedly reduced when compared to the other eye (this is a very robust sign of dendritic ulceration)
- Visual acuity is often mildly reduced
- Dendrite can be seen on corneal examination. Although corneal examination with the naked eye can sometimes detect a dendritic ulcer, fluorescein staining and suitable magnification make this task much easier. The ulcer has a branching pattern (Figure 16.8).

treatment some patients will develop corneal scarring with blood vessel ingrowth that can decrease visual acuity (Figure 16.7). The symptoms are very similar to those of iritis, although watering is often more marked. In the first day or two the pain can be quite mild.

Action

Acyclovir (Zovirax®) ointment is prescribed five times a day. This should be under specialist supervision, but initial treatment may be started in primary care as soon as the diagnosis is made (The preparation for skin application is not suitable). The ulcers usually heal in 1–2 weeks without complication. Recurrence is common, and is treated in the same way.

If treated with steroid drops, ulcers rapidly expand to become geographic ulcers. These are difficult to heal and often lead to corneal scarring with decreased visual acuity.

Figure 16.8 Dendritic ulcer stained with fluorescein and viewed under blue light. Reproduced with permission from *Clinical Ophthalmology* by J. Kanski, 1999.

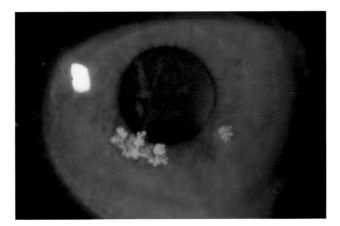

Acute glaucoma

Acute glaucoma occurs in small eyes where space within the eye is reduced by an enlarging lens. The lens of the eye increases in size throughout life, but in small eyes (usually hypermetropes) this increase in size shallows the anterior chamber and can eventually lead to blockage of the trabecular meshwork by peripheral iris (Figure 16.9). The condition is almost unknown in patients under 55 years of age because the lens is not big enough to cause trouble before this time. The drainage route for aqueous becomes blocked off, and the pressure within the eye steadily rises as production of aqueous continues unabated. Pain, located not in the eye but in the eyebrow, is the overriding feature, and may cause nausea or vomiting.

Figure 16.9 Comparison between a normal and a small eye demonstrating a shallow anterior chamber and the resulting narrow access to the trabecular meshwork.

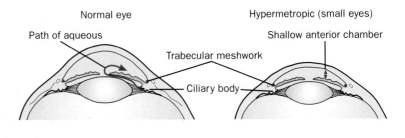

Normal eye

Hypermetropic (small eyes)

Path of aqueous

Shallow anterior chamber

Trabecular meshwork

Ciliary body

Findings

The amount of redness of the eye can vary, but vision is usually decreased. Acute glaucoma, like iritis and dendritic ulcer, is often misdiagnosed as conjunctivitis. Also in common with iritis and dendritic ulcer, there is no history of mucopurulent discharge and without appropriate treatment the condition gets worse every day.

- Visual acuity is usually reduced and the cornea has a ground-glass appearance
- All patients have a mid-dilated, often oval-shaped, pupil that does not react to light or accommodation (Figure 16.10)
- On digital palpation, the eyeball is stony hard compared with the unaffected eye. Bilateral cases are almost unheard of and so it is possible to compare the pressure in each eye.

Action

Patients should be referred immediately so that the intraocular pressure – typically between 45 and 60 mmHg – can be reduced. Once intraocular pressure has been controlled, a long-term cure can be affected by fashioning an alternative route for aqueous drainage (laser iridotomy) or by removal of the offending structure, the lens, in an identical procedure to a cataract operation. Cases in which there has been a delay in diagnosis can be refractory to treatment, and may require a trabeculectomy.

Figure 16.10 Acute angle closure glaucoma. Note the mid-dilated pupil and corneal haze obscuring any iris detail.

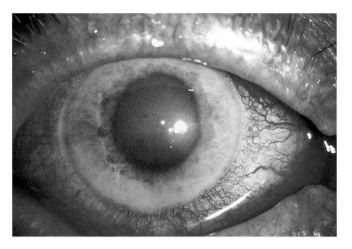

RED EYE WITHOUT SIGNIFICANT PAIN OR PUS

Episcleritis

Episcleritis is common and self limiting, typically affecting young adults. Patients usually notice a discrete area of redness associated with mild discomfort, and the eye is tender to touch (Figure 16.11). There is no history of stickiness. Symptoms resolve in 1–2 weeks, but a weak topical cortico-steroid drop four times a day will hasten resolution. If the condition is very painful it is likely that the diagnosis is scleritis, in which case the patient will need to be referred for treatment and investigation for an underlying cause.

Figure 16.11 Episcleritis. Reproduced with permission from *Clinical Ophthalmology* by J. Kanski, 1999.

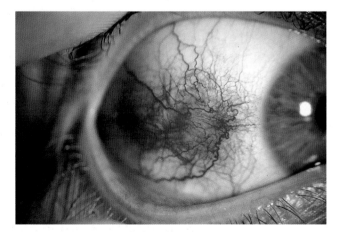

Viral conjunctivitis

Viral conjunctivitis is caused by adenoviruses and is usually bilateral. Patients develop a watering red eye but there is no mucopurulent discharge initially, although secondary bacterial infection may occur. The eye is usually uncomfortable and photophobic, and a history of a recent cold is typical. Follicles are seen in the lower conjunctival fornix, and preauricular lymphadenopathy is often present.

The condition is self limiting, resolving within a couple of weeks. It is infectious and tends to occur in epidemics, with whole families affected. No treatment is required unless it is severe, in which case referral is indicated.

Subconjunctival haemorrhage

Subconjunctival haemorrhages can occur spontaneously after vomiting or post-trauma – including vigorous rubbing of the eyes (Figure 16.12). If patients are on warfarin, it is prudent to check that they are not consuming an excessive dose. The condition is self-limiting and will resolve untreated in a week or so.

Figure 16.12 Subconjunctival haemorrhage. As opposed to other types of red eye, the conjunctival vessels are not engorged but are merely covered with a film of blood.

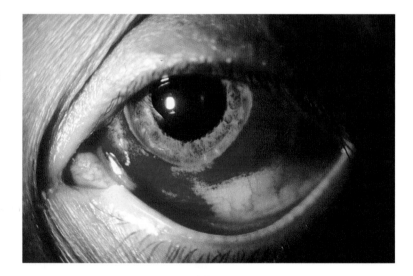

PAINFUL EYES

On examination the eye is often red, and it is worth excluding diagnoses such as acute glaucoma or corneal ulcer (both bacterial and dendritic).

History

Important features of the history include (Figure 16.13):

● Chronicity
● Trauma
    A foreign body entering the eye (stick or fingernail, wind-borne or industrial objects)
● Contact lens wear
● Ultraviolet light exposure
    Snow blindness
    Welding flash ('arc eye')
    Sun lamp
● Sudden pain on waking.

Figure 16.13 Identifying the cause of a painful eye.

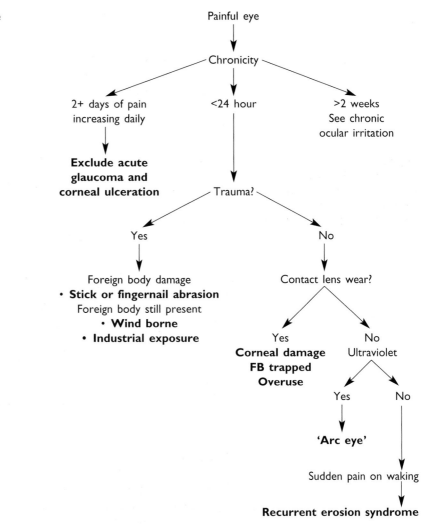

Examination

This focuses on the cornea and occasionally requires the top lid to be everted in the hunt for a hidden foreign body. Suspicion of acute glaucoma or corneal ulceration can be confirmed in the usual way. Foreign bodies stuck to the cornea can be seen by direct examination, and fluorescein staining easily highlights breaks in the corneal surface caused by trauma or ultraviolet exposure.

Corneal abrasion

In corneal abrasion, the superficial corneal epithelium is removed. Frequent perpetrators of the crime are children's fingernails, Yucca plants, gardening canes, and clumsy contact lens owners. There is intense pain and lacrimation with blepharospasm (eyelids squeezed tight shut) to the extent that local anaesthetic drops are often needed to allow proper examination. The patient often describes a foreign body sensation in the eye.

> **Findings**
>
> Once the lids are open the eye is usually red, and fluorescein staining reveals the reason why (Figure 16.14).

Figure 16.14 Large corneal abrasion stained with fluorescein and viewed under blue light. Reproduced with permission from *Clinical Ophthalmology* by J. Kanski, 1999.

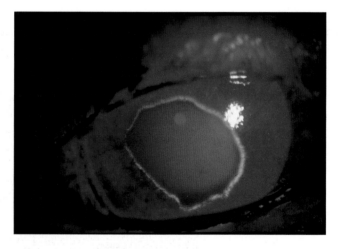

> *Action*
>
> Topical anaesthetics should only be used for temporary relief of pain while the eye is being examined, as they inhibit corneal epithelial regrowth. After this, cyclopentolate drops should be used. These drops paralyse the ciliary muscle, whose spasm causes some of the pain. Topical chloramphenicol ointment provides lubrication and some antibiotic prophylaxis against infection. Finally, an eye pad for 24 hours usually allows the defect to heal successfully. If the eye does not feel markedly better after this time or a white/yellow infiltrate appears in the region of the abrasion, the patient should be referred urgently for management of a possible corneal ulcer.

Foreign body

The majority of foreign bodies are wind-borne or industrial.

Wind-borne foreign bodies

In these cases, a piece of grit enters the eye, usually on a windy day. Most particles are washed out of the eye by the tear film; however, if a foreign body sensation persists for more than a few minutes the particle of grit has become trapped under the top lid and each movement of the top lid causes scratching of the corneal surface. Patients complain of a foreign body sensation associated with lacrimation.

Findings

- The eye may be red, and corneal staining with fluorescein reveals why – vertical scratches are seen on the corneal surface (Figure 16.15)
- In many cases no foreign body will found as it has eventually been washed out of the eye by the profuse lacrimation.

Figure 16.15 Scratches on the cornea caused by a subtarsal foreign body.

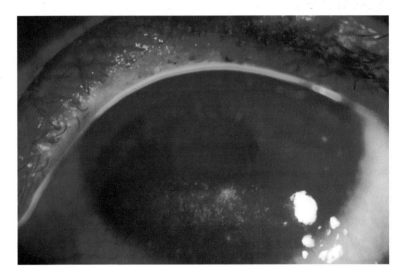

Action

The top lid needs to be everted, as this is where the foreign body will be if there is one to be found. The foreign body is often quite small and can be easily removed with a dry cotton bud. Further treatment with chloramphenicol eye ointment to guard against infection while the epithelium heals, along with an eye pad for 24 hours, complete the treatment. Following this, the ointment should be used four times a day for 3 days.

Industrial foreign bodies

In these cases, the patient was typically carrying out some kind of work – for example, grinding a piece of metal. The increased velocity and mass of the object (usually a fragment of metal or welding slag) mean that it becomes embedded in the corneal surface. The symptoms are the same as above. Interestingly, grinding never causes penetration of the eye because the fragments are not travelling fast enough. However, a history of 'metal on metal' (e.g. chiselling a ball bearing) should arouse suspicion of a penetrating eye injury, because these activities do cause fragments to travel fast enough to penetrate the eye.

> **Findings**
>
> The metal fragments are seen embedded in the cornea, and are usually visible to the naked eye although fluorescein staining can be of help.

> **Action**
>
> Foreign bodies can be relatively easily flipped out using the tip of a hypodermic needle (Figure 16.16). Further treatment is identical to that described above. If the injury is several hours old a 'rust ring' leaches out into the surrounding cornea, leaving a brown halo once the foreign body has been removed (Figure 16.17). If a rust ring remains in the cornea after removal of the foreign body, the patient should be given chloramphenicol eye ointment (this loosens the rust ring) along with an eye pad and send them to an eye casualty the next day for removal of the rust ring.

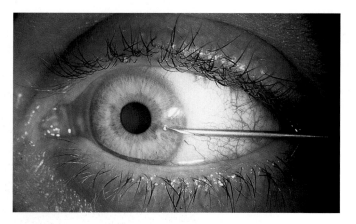

Figure 16.16 Metallic foreign body. Removal should first be attempted using a cotton bud under topical anaesthesia. If this fails, a needle may succeed.

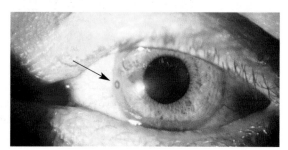

Figure 16.17 Corneal rust ring.

Contact lens problems

Contact lenses form a protective barrier over the cornea and, because of this, patients while wearing contact lenses are unaware of corneal mishaps and do not complain until the lens has been removed. Two common problems are overuse (in particular, wearing lenses only designed for day wear all night) and foreign bodies getting behind the contact lens and scratching the cornea. Examination findings and treatment are the same as for other types of foreign body. Any contact lenses should be removed during treatment, and should only be replaced once all pain and redness have settled and the lenses have been cleaned thoroughly.

Ultraviolet light exposure

Exposure to UV light typically causes an intense bout of pain, photophobia and lacrimation about 6 hours after the event. Usually the condition follows arc welding or using a sun-bed without eye protection. After topical anaesthesia and fluorescein staining, small widespread epithelial erosions can be seen covering the cornea (Figure 16.18). Treatment with a pad and chloramphenicol ointment along with suitable pain relief brings about a speedy recovery.

Figure 16.18 Punctate epithelial erosions stained with fluorescein and viewed under blue light. Reproduced with permission from *Clinical Ophthalmology* by J. Kanski, 1999.

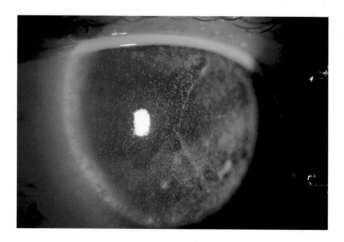

Recurrent erosion syndrome

This condition has a very specific history. Patients complain of a sudden pain that occurs immediately on opening the eyes in the morning. They may also give a history of previous corneal injury, and liken the pain to that experienced during the initial injury. Examination shows a corneal defect best seen using fluorescein staining, and the position of the defect corresponds to the area of the initial injury. The condition occurs due to a failure of normal adhesion of the corneal epithelium to the corneal stroma during healing of the original injury. Initial treatment with chloramphenicol and an eye pad is effective in controlling symptoms; however, recurrences are common and referral to the eye department may well be required for further management. There, debridement of loose epithelium and multiple stromal puncture with a hypodermic needle or in some cases excimer laser photoablation are required in order to persuade the epithelium to heal correctly.

Chronic ocular irritation

The complaint of chronically uncomfortable eyes is a common one. Itchiness, grittiness, burning and stinging are the common symptoms. The eyes may also show a degree of redness. It is usually apparent that the patient's condition is not serious, but the discomfort is clearly annoying. The condition has typically already run for some weeks, months or even years!

History

Different causes of uncomfortable eyes are more likely at various ages. In the table, the age bands quoted are approximate and there may be considerable overlap: a patient aged 35 years with a systemic disease such as rheumatoid arthritis may have significantly dry eyes.

Age (years)	Condition
18–50	Allergic eye disease
	Blepharitis
	Drug toxicity
50+ years	Blepharitis
	Drug toxicity
	Dry eyes
	Entropion
	Trichiasis

Although all the symptoms may appear together, the dominant complaint can point toward a specific diagnosis:

- Itchiness – allergy
- Grittiness – dry eye
- Stinging/burning – blepharitis.

Other details in the history are also worth enquiring about:

- Atopy – hay fever/rhinitis/asthma/eczema
- Systemic disease – rheumatoid arthritis
- Previous meibomium cysts/styes
- Current eye drop usage.

Examination

This will focus on:

- Face – looking for
    Rosacea (patients are very prone to blepharitis)
    Seborrhoea (patients are very prone to blepharitis)
    Eczema (patients are prone to allergic eye disease)
    Proptosis (very occasionally thyroid eye disease can present with chronic ocular irritation)
- Eyelids – looking for
    Blepharitis
    Entropion
    Trichiasis (misdirected eyelashes rubbing on the cornea)
- Conjunctiva – follicles in the fornix are suggestive of an allergic reaction
- Cornea (with fluorescein staining)– corneal erosions

As with the acutely red eye, it is worth making sure that the eye or eyes are not proptosed. The finding of proptosis is subjective, but if found is highly significant and demands early referral for further investigation.

Allergic eye disease

The basic types are:

- Allergic rhinoconjunctivitis
    Seasonal (hay fever)
    Perennial
- Atopic.

Allergic rhinoconjunctivitis

> **Findings**
> - Patients typically present with transient attacks of itchy, slightly red, watery eyes, which may be associated with sneezing and a snuffly nose
> - There are follicles in the lower conjunctiva (see Chapter 16).

Patients suffering from seasonal or perennial allergic eye disease frequently experience associated nasal symptoms; hence the term allergic rhinoconjunctivitis.

Seasonal conjunctivitis is triggered by sensitivity to pollens during the hay fever season, while perennial allergic conjunctivitis is triggered by allergy to common household allergens such as house-dust mites or animal dander. Patients with perennial allergic eye disease are affected all year round, although the condition is often worse in the winter because central heating creates convection currents that circulate otherwise dormant allergens.

> **Action**
>
> Most cases are successfully managed in the community with mast cell stabilizers such as sodium cromoglycate or Iodoxamide drops four times a day. In the case of seasonal sufferers, treatment should be started a month before the hay fever season begins.

Atopic allergic eye disease

This is potentially sight threatening, and fortunately much less common than seasonal and perennial allergy. The local ophthalmologist manages most patients. Eczema is often present on the face, with thickened and fissured eyelids. Chronic staphylococcal infection is common. Even with steroid therapy corneal ulceration, scarring and vascularization may ultimately decrease vision.

Blepharitis

Blepharitis (from the Greek, *blepharon*: eyelid) is very common, and is usually bilateral and symmetrical. A mixture of chronic staphylococcal infection and abnormal oil secretions from the meibomium glands gives rise to chronic inflammation of the eyelids and ocular irritation. An unstable tear film occurs in many cases, resulting in an overlay of dry eye symptoms (see below). The main symptoms are usually worse in the mornings, and are characterized by a relapsing and remitting course:

- Burning
- Crusting and redness of lid margins
- Grittiness.

> **Findings**
>
> - Acne rosacea of the face or seborrhoeic dermatitis affecting the scalp, nasolabial folds or brow may be apparent (Figure 17.1)
> - The lid margins are variably red, often with teleiangectatic blood vessels and, in advanced cases, scarring and notching of the lid margin
> - The eyelashes may be greasy and stuck together (Figure 17.2) or have hard scales centred on the base of the lashes (Figure 17.3); the latter suggests staphylococcal infection
> - Oil globules maybe apparent at the entrance to the meibomium glands, and finger pressure on the lid expresses more oil (Figue 17.4).
> - The meibomium glands may be blocked with semi-solid secretions (Figure 17.5) causing underlying chronic inflammation. Finger pressure on the lid just below the lash line may express a tube of viscid tooth-paste-like material (sometimes referred to as 'meibomianitis').

Figure 17.1 Rosacea facies.

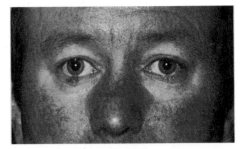

Figure 17.2 Blepharitis with greasy stuck-together lashes. Reproduced with permission from *Clinical Ophthalmology* by J. Kanski, 1999.

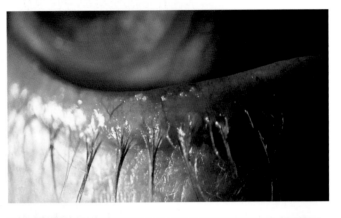

Figure 17.3 Blepharitis with scales at the lash bases. Reproduced with permission from *Clinical Ophthalmology* by J. Kanski, 1999.

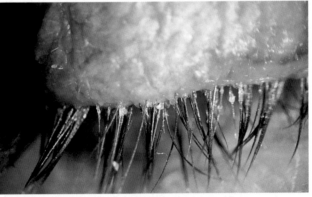

Figure 17.4 Blepharitis with capping of the meibomium gland orifices with oil. Reproduced with permission from *Clinical Ophthalmology* by J. Kanski, 1999.

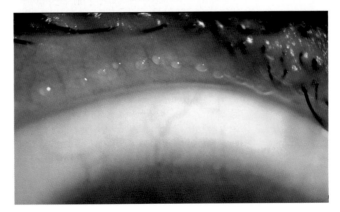

Figure 17.5 Blepharitis with semi-solid secretions blocking the meibomium gland orifices. Reproduced with permission from *Clinical Ophthalmology* by J. Kanski, 1999.

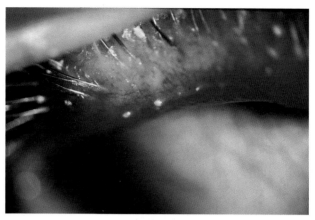

Action

Treatment can usually improve the patient's comfort and help control the symptoms. However, cure is not possible. Eyelid hygiene is the mainstay of treatment. It is important to keep the eyelid clean by removing all lash crusts and washing the eyelid margins with dilute baby shampoo (1 : 4 parts water, using a cotton bud or face cloth) to remove any irritant oils. Expressing any meibomium secretions beforehand will also help. Warm compresses such as a hot flannel or a facial steamer will also help to open pores before cleaning. Initially this cleaning regimen should be undertaken twice a day, but once the condition is under control a couple of times a week should suffice.

Those cases with crusts among the lashes will also benefit from rubbing fusidic acid (fucithalmic®) ointment into the lash area once the eyelids have been cleaned.

Cases with blocked meibomium glands (meibomianitis) or rosacea/seborrhoea benefit from systemic tetracycline treatment. Oxytetracycline 250 mg four times a day or minocycline 100 mg once a day for a period of 12 weeks often produces improvement in both the eyelid and facial skin.

Many patients also experience dry eye symptoms, and so tear film supplements are helpful.

Complications

- Meibomium cyst – blockage of the gland entrance leads to stagnation of sebaceous secretions and chronic inflammation (see Chapter 13)
- Styes – staphylococcal infection may spread to the lash root (see Chapter 13)
- Marginal keratitis – this is a hypersensitivity reaction to staphylococcal antigens, causing a white peripheral corneal ulcer (Figure 17.6)
- Trichiasis – aberrant lash growth can result from scarred lids, leading to permanent cornea/lash touch.

Figure 17.6 Marginal keratitis. These ulcers are benign in nature but are difficult to distinguish from a more serious bacterial ulcer, and so are best reviewed in the eye casualty department. Reproduced with permission from *Clinical Ophthalmology* by J. Kanski, 1999.

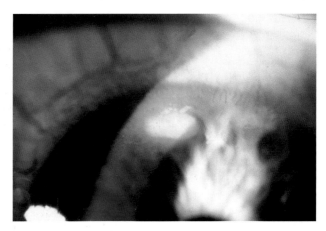

All of the above are more common amongst patients with rosacea or seborrhoea.

Dry eyes

With advancing age, conjunctival goblet cells are lost and dryness of the eyes can result. The classic symptom is grittiness. Patients often complain that it feels as if they have sand in the eye. Reflex watering (from the main lacrimal gland) may also occur, causing puzzlement amongst patients when you inform them of your diagnosis.

Patients with rheumatoid arthritis can suffer from dry eyes as part of Sjögren's syndrome. In some patients it is very severe, leading to great discomfort and even corneal perforation.

Findings

- In most cases there is nothing to see, and the diagnosis is based on the classic symptom complex and exclusion of other conditions causing a chronically irritable eye
- In advanced cases, the cornea will show tiny punctate staining with fluorescein (Figure 17.7).

Figure 17.7 Dry eyes. Punctate epithelial erosions stained with fluorescein. Reproduced with permission from *Clinical Ophthalmology* by J. Kanski, 1999.

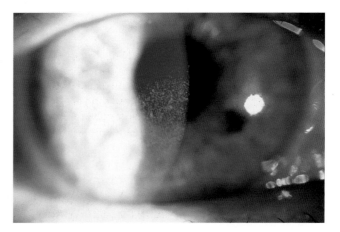

Entropion

Findings

- Inspection of the eyelids reveals an inverted lower lid (Figure 17.8).

Entropion is an inversion of the lower lid that causes the eyelashes to rub on the cornea. It results from stretching of the tendons and muscles of the lower lid, and is generally seen in the elderly.

The condition causes discomfort, and the patient may complain of a foreign body sensation. Secondary bacterial conjunctivitis may also occur intermittently.

Figure 17.8 Entropion.

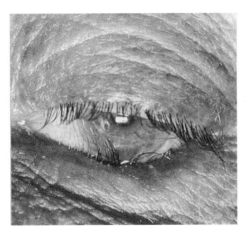

Action

Surgical correction is required. Everting sutures are simple and effective, and they have the advantage that they can be placed in an outpatient setting as well as in a nursing home setting if the patient cannot be moved. The procedure is highly successful, but the condition may recur. More complex eyelid procedures exist for recurrent cases.

Trichiasis

Aberrant lashes can grow backwards and abrade the cornea, causing irritation (Figure 17.9).

Figure 17.9 Trichiasis. Patients report a foreign body sensation, and may already be periodically plucking out the offending lash. Reproduced with permission from *Clinical Ophthalmology* by J. Kanski, 1999.

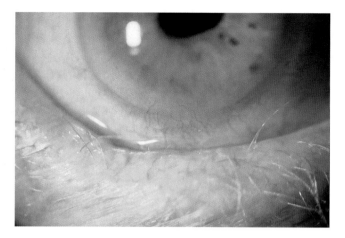

Findings

- A misdirected lash is seen on inspection of the eyelids.

Action

In the community, patients may deal with the problem themselves by periodic plucking of the offending lash. The infirm may ask a relative or an appropriate nurse to do the honours. Treatment in the eye department has two approaches to cure the problem:

- Electrolysis/laser/cryotherapy of the lash root, although recurrence of the aberrant lash is very common
- Wedge excision of the eyelid margin containing the offending lash, which gives a permanent cure.

Findings

- Pain on instillation of drops
- Photophobia
- Red conjunctiva
- Punctate erosions on fluorescein staining.

Action

The offending drops should be stopped. If continued medication is required, unpreserved drops should be prescribed.

Drug toxicity

Drops these days do not come in brown glass bottles with short shelf lives. The reason for this is the addition of preservatives, which extend the shelf life of each bottle up to a month. Unfortunately, these preservatives can be toxic to the eye. Patients on long-term medication (say for dry eyes or glaucoma) may complain of ocular irritation and stinging on instillation of the drops. This is not a good sign, and usually indicates intolerance to preservatives. In severe cases (some patients persevere with the drops despite the pain) the conjunctiva is red and angry. Toxicity-induced corneal erosions cause gritty pain and photophobia, and can lead to the temptation to diagnose severe dry eye with the prescription of yet more drops.

Thyroid eye disease

Hyperthyroidism in the acute phase can very rarely present with chronically irritable eyes. The patient complains of swollen, puffy lids with irritation and watering eyes. Examination confirms these findings, as well as a red eye and usually a degree of proptosis (see Chapter 12). The patient is exhibiting acute thyroid eye disease, and a history of weight loss and tremor are usually present. Referral to the hospital for control of the thyroid gland as well as treatment of the eyes is required (see Chapter 21).

Part IV

Trauma

Trauma

Trivial trauma, such as foreign bodies and corneal abrasions, is dealt with in Chapter 16. More severe trauma can be categorized, depending on the history, as:

● Chemical injury
● Blunt injury
● Sharp injury.

CHEMICAL INJURY

Chemical injuries tend to occur as part of an assault or an industrial accident. Strong acids and alkalis are extremely toxic to the eye, and are notorious for causing blindness in the affected eyes. Occult strong alkali is in common industrial use, in the form of cement and plaster. These compounds contain calcium hydroxide (lime) and can cause severe damage to the eyes; they strip off the corneal epithelium and also kill the stem cells from which replacement epithelium derives. Instead of epithelial regeneration, healing occurs via vascular ingrowth and scarring (Figure 18.1). Vascularization

Figure 18.1 Severe alkali injury. The eye is blind due to corneal vascularization and scar formation. The prospects for a successful corneal transplant are poor.

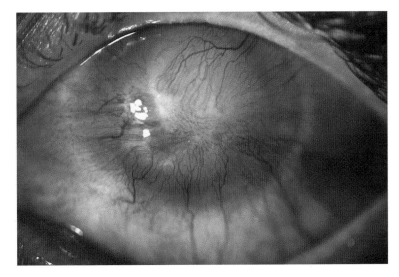

of the cornea carries a poor prognosis for corneal transplantation, and this form of treatment for scarred corneas usually fails.

> **Action**
>
> The mainstay of treatment is immediate and copious irrigation with neutral fluids such as water or normal saline. This should occur as soon as possible, and last for 20 minutes or more in the case of strong compounds. Any loose material such as cement particles should be removed from the eye. Emergency referral to the eye department should only occur after thorough initial irrigation.

BLUNT INJURY

This is the commonest type of injury and occurs in all walks of life from common assault to sporting injury. The size of the offensive object determines to a large extent the types of injury sustained:

- Objects larger than the bony orbit include, for example
    Fists
    Tennis balls
- Objects smaller than the bony orbit include, for example
    Squash balls/shuttlecocks
    Elastic luggage straps
    Champagne corks
    Airgun pellets.

Objects larger than the bony orbit

These tend to cause large periocular haematomas with or without lid lacerations (Figure 18.2). If the force is consider-

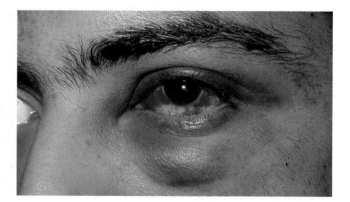

Figure 18.2 Periocular haematoma with subconjunctival haemorrhage. Reproduced with permission from *Clinical Ophthalmology* by J. Kanski, 1999.

Figure 18.3 Laceration of the lid margin. Reproduced with permission from *Clinical Ophthalmology* by J. Kanski, 1999.

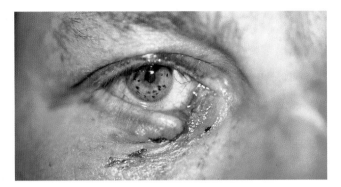

able, a blow-out fracture of the orbital floor may occur (see Chapter 10). Ripping injuries caused by individual fingers can disrupt the lid margin (Figure 18.3). However, the eye itself is often protected by the bony orbit and sustains little damage.

> **Action**
>
> Lid lacerations require referral, as a precise primary repair is needed if lid function is to be restored. Double vision is suggestive of a blow-out fracture, and this requires specialist intervention. Mild haematomas probably do not require referral, but it is worth remembering that retinal detachment is a significant complication that may occur in the days or weeks following injury.

Objects smaller than the bony orbit

Smaller objects can gain access to the surface of the eye unimpeded by the bony orbit. 'Direct hits' cause a compression injury of the globe. The commonest feature is a hyphaema (Figure 18.4) following rupture of iris blood vessels. Rupture of the iris sphincter is also common, and presents as a dilated and unreactive pupil. The patient is usually fully conscious, and this sign should not be confused with 'blowing a pupil' associated with subdural haematomas, where the patient is generally unconscious.

> **Action**
>
> A whole litany of injuries to the eye can occur, including rupture of the globe, and therefore all patients are best referred for assessment, especially if there is a decrease in the visual acuity. Post-traumatic retinal detachment is common. Airgun pellets usually glance off the side of the sclera and pass into the orbit behind the globe. If they are causing no harm, they are usually left alone. Injury to the iris root may cause scarring of the trabecular meshwork and glaucoma. This may occur as late as 10 years after the initial incident, and so long-term monitoring of intraocular pressure by the optician is indicated.

Figure 18.4 Hyphaema. Blood in the anterior chamber will precipitate, and form a fluid level inferiorly. Movement will stir up the blood cells and reduce visual acuity.

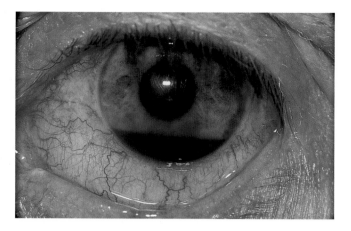

SHARP INJURY

Again, the size and shape of the offending object is likely to dictate the type of injury. Large objects may only cause laceration of the orbital skin and eyelids, while small objects are likely to penetrate the globe. A history of hammering metal on metal (e.g. chiselling a ball bearing) is likely to produce sharp metal fragments travelling at very high velocity. These are notorious for causing penetrating injuries and intraocular foreign bodies. If the penetrating wound is big enough intraocular pressure is lost and the anterior chamber collapses, often with prolapse of iris tissue (Figure 18.5).

> *Action*
>
> Urgent referral for assessment and repair is indicated. In general, penetrating injuries carry a poor prognosis for future vision. Occasionally the eye is so badly disrupted that primary removal of the eye is indicated.

Figure 18.5 Iris prolapse is clear sign of penetrating eye injury.

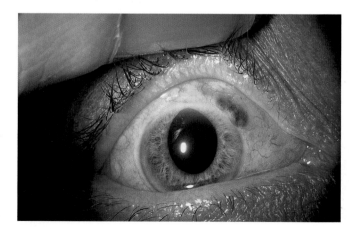

SYMPATHETIC OPHTHALMITIS

This is an extremely rare uveitis that affects both eyes after previous penetrating trauma to one eye. It develops between 2 weeks and 1 year after the initial trauma and, if not spotted by the ophthalmologist, can have disastrous effects on the vision of the good eye. Patients complain of blurred vision in both eyes. The penetrating trauma probably exposes the immune system to previously unrecognized uveal proteins that are then attacked in both eyes, having been assumed to be foreign.

ARTIFICIAL EYES

Removal of an eye is occasionally necessary after trauma, but is also sometimes necessary to relieve suffering in patients with blind and painful eyes. These eyes are usually the final result of failed treatment for a myriad of chronic ocular conditions. A good cosmetic outcome is best achieved by replacing lost volume in the socket with an orbital implant. The extraocular muscles are then attached to the implant to allow synchronous movement of the implant with the other eye (Figure 18.6). Convincing eye movements can be achieved in this way (Figure 18.7).

Figure 18.6 Orbital implant with a glass prosthesis inserted into the conjunctival sac.

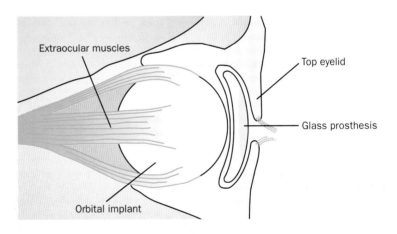

Extraocular muscles

Top eyelid

Glass prosthesis

Orbital implant

Figure 18.7 The artificial eye is the one on the left!

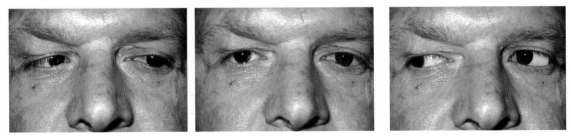

Part V

Chronic watering eyes

Chronic watering eyes

This can be due to either an overproduction of tears or poor drainage of normal amounts of tears.

- Overproduction
    - Allergy
    - Dry eye
    - Mucus fishing
    - Entropion
- Poor drainage
    - Ectropion
    - Blocked nasolacrimal system.

A combination of history and examination will point the way to the most likely diagnosis. Allergy is usually obvious, with its associated itchiness and rhinitis.

OVERPRODUCTION

Dry eye

One paradox patients can find difficult is the complaint of a watering eye with a diagnosis of dry eye. The explanation is that dry eye results from decreased basal secretion of tears from the conjunctival goblet cells, and this dryness causes reflex watering of the main lacrimal gland. Patients will also experience gritty eyes, which are typical of the condition. The cornea, on staining with fluorescein, may show punctate erosions (see Chapter 17). Indeed, any condition that causes chronic damage to the corneal epithelium will induce watering, and this is the case with entropion (see Chapter 17), where the inturning lashes abrade the cornea. This diagnosis is confirmed on examination of the lower lids.

Mucus fishing

This is a little recognized practice that some patients indulge in, often started after a bout of conjunctivitis that is now long

> **Action**
>
> Patients must be persuaded to sit on their hands for a week, and their symptoms may then miraculously disappear.

forgotten. These patients daily remove mucus from the corner of the eye, or even from the lower conjunctival sac. This practice has two consequences; the first is damage to the conjunctival epithelium, which induces watering, and the second is the production of more mucus to try and protect the damaged epithelium. This, of course, is picked out the next day, and the process is repeated.

POOR DRAINAGE

Ectropion

> **Action**
>
> Routine referral for correction of ectropion is indicated. If the condition is long-standing, the punctum may have shrunk in size and also need enlarging.

With age (and constant rubbing) the eyelid tendons weaken, causing laxity. This may lead to eversion of the whole of the bottom lid or, in some cases, just the medial end. The lower punctum is located at the medial end of the lid and, if it is not snug up against the globe, watering will occur. When the whole lid is everted, ectropion (Figure 19.1) is not a taxing diagnosis; however, if only the medial end is affected the signs can be subtle (Figure 19.2).

Figure 19.1 Ectropion. A secondary conjunctivitis is not uncommon.

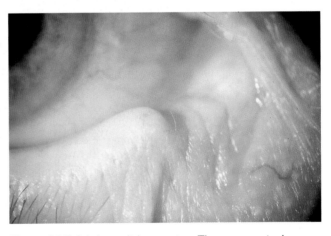

Figure 19.2 Subtle medial ectropion. The punctum is drawn away from the eyeball. Reproduced with permission from *Clinical Ophthalmology* by J. Kanski, 1999.

Blocked nasolacrimal system

Once tears have collected at the puncti, they drain via the canaliculi to the nasolacrimal duct. This is situated underneath the medial canthal tendon at the junction between the nose and orbit. The duct enters a bony canal in the orbit and descends finally to open into the nose (Figure 19.3). Blockage

Figure 19.3 Anatomy of the lacrimal system. Reproduced with permission from *Clinical Ophthalmology* by J. Kanski, 1999.

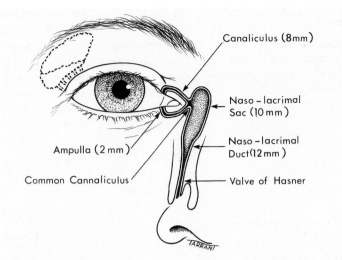

Figure 19.4 Acute dacryocystitis. Reproduced with permission from *Clinical Ophthalmology* by J. Kanski, 1999.

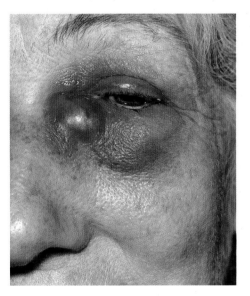

Action

Acute infections require oral and occasionally intravenous broad-spectrum antibiotics. Some require lancing to effect a rapid cure. Other non-acute cases should be referred for possible surgery. Dacryocysto-rhinostomy (DCR) is the mainstay operation, and can be performed via either an external skin or an internal intranasal approach.

of the system causes continual watering, which occurs both indoors and outdoors. Occasionally a stagnant pool of mucus collects in the duct (mucocoele) and white viscid material can be expressed from the lower punctum with pressure on the medial canthal tendon. Acute infection of this collection leads to a painful abscess ('dacryocystitis') on the side of the nose

Dacryocystorhinostomy

By removing part of the lateral wall of the nose it is possible to anastomose the nasal epithelium with the epithelium lining the nasolacrimal sac. In this way a new passage for the tears is fashioned that bypasses any blockages in the narrow nasolacrimal duct.

Most cases are operated upon under general anaesthetic, with perhaps a single night's stay in hospital. Around 80–90 per cent of cases are successful.

Part VI

The optician's letter

The optician's letter

One of the common presentations of eye conditions to the general practitioner is via the optician's letter. Many of the patients have consulted the optician routinely, and during these visits the optician may have spotted conditions that patients don't complain about. Others consult because of blurred vision, and in this group the optician commonly sees patients with cataract and macular degeneration (see Chapter 7).

CONDITIONS PATIENTS DON'T COMPLAIN ABOUT

By their very nature these conditions are asymptomatic and are usually only found on routine ophthalmic examination at an optician's visit:

● Chronic simple glaucoma
● Pigmented retinal lesions.

GLAUCOMA

The glaucomas are a group of ocular diseases that damage the optic nerve, causing characteristic cupping and visual field defects (scotomas). In most cases this damage results from raised intraocular pressure. Opticians have the equipment to measure all of these parameters, and if an abnormal result is turned up on routine examination they will refer patients for further investigation.

Action

The diagnosis of glaucoma is complex and requires the skills of an ophthalmologist (except for acute glaucoma, of course). A non-urgent referral is indicated. By far and away the majority of these patients will be discharged, as further testing reveals no abnormality; however, occasional patients will be kept under review because one of the following is diagnosed:

• Chronic simple glaucoma
• Ocular hypertension
• Normal tension glaucoma.

Chronic simple glaucoma

In a few cases (secondary and chronic closed angle glaucoma) the cause of the raised pressure is discovered; however, in most cases it is not and the eye appears normal. This is known as chronic simple glaucoma or open angle glaucoma, and it affects 0.5 per cent of the population over 40 years old.

The central visual field is not affected until the condition is very advanced, and so chronic simple glaucoma is generally asymptomatic despite peripheral field loss. In the same way, consider that most people are unaware of their physiological blind spot, which is of considerable size and only 15° off the axis of fixation. This is why opticians actively need to screen for glaucoma.

Diagnosis

Diagnosis is based on assessment of the optic disc and visual field as well as measurement of the intraocular pressure, and the following will be seen:

- High intraocular pressure
- Optic disc cupping
- Typical scotomas in the visual field.

Intraocular pressure: The gold standard for measuring pressure is Goldmann contact tonometry (Figure 20.1). The upper end for normal intraocular pressure is traditionally 21 mmHg.

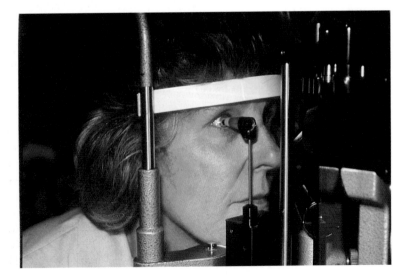

Figure 20.1 Goldmann contact tonometry. This method often takes lower readings than the methods used by opticians, and explains why abnormal readings found by the optician are not always confirmed in the eye department.

Figure 20.2 Early glaucomatous damage may present as notching of the neuroretinal rim, especially at the top or bottom of the disc.

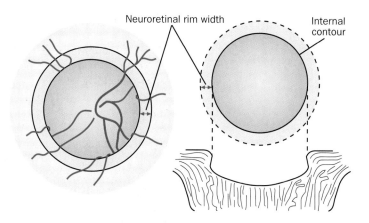

Neuroretinal rim width   Internal contour

Optic disc assessment: This is very difficult because of the infinite variety of normal optic discs. The main visible sign is erosion of the neuroretinal rim (Figure 20.2) causing a larger central cup. As the disease progresses, the neuroretinal rim is slowly eroded until there is little or no rim left (Figure 20.3).

Figure 20.3 End stage glaucomatous cupping. Note the wide central cup and thin neuroretinal rim.

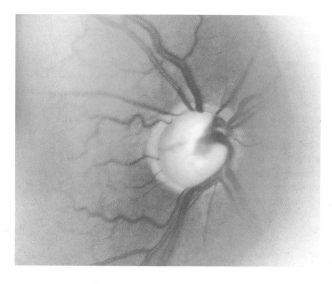

However, some patients have large optic discs with large central cups but normal-sized neuroretinal rims (Figure 20.4). The key to diagnosis is to look at the neuroretinal rim of the disc and check that it is of reasonable width with a smooth internal contour.

Visual fields and retinal anatomy: Loss of nerve fibres in the neuroretinal rim described above results in visual field loss. The pattern of field loss is determined by retinal anatomy.

Figure 20.4 Some patients have large optic discs with large central cups but normal-sized neuroretinal rims. The optic discs of these patients are normal and are known as physiologically cupped discs.

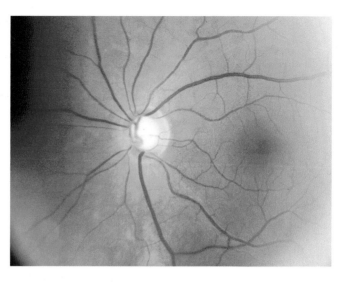

The macula contains the highest density of optic nerve fibres, and these occupy a disproportionate amount of room at the optic disc (most of the temporal side). Fibres subserving the rest of the temporal retina are squeezed into the superior and inferior portions of the optic disc, and have to arch around the macular fibres to reach their destinations (Figure 20.5).

Figure 20.5 The upper and lower areas of the disc are most susceptible to glaucomatous damage, and so the typical field defect seen is an 'arcuate' (arching) scotoma. With advanced disease the macular fibres become damaged as well, leaving the patient blind.

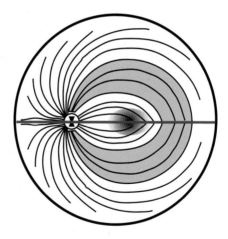

There are several methods for measuring visual fields, but most ophthalmologists use the Humphrey machine. This machine is computer driven and automatically monitors a patient's performance. A visual field test requires the patient to maintain concentration for periods of up to 10 minutes. Age and coexisting disease, such as cataract and age-related macular degeneration, mean that approximately 20 per cent of the population are unable to complete the test satisfactorily. Clinical decisions must then be taken on the appearance of the optic disc and the intraocular pressure reading alone.

Secondary glaucoma and chronic angle closure glaucoma

Occasionally the cause of the raised intraocular pressure is known. The reasons vary:

- Increased resistance to outflow
    Post-traumatic scarring of the trabecular meshwork
    Use of corticosteroid preparations in the eye or on the eyelid skin
    Trabeculitis caused by herpes zoster infection
- Blockage of the outflow system
    Blood cells (post-hyphema)
    Inflammatory cells (uveitis)
    Amyloid material (pseudoexfoliation syndrome)
    Pigment cells (pigment dispersion syndrome)
- Inadequate access to the drainage angle
    Chronic angle closure
    New vessels in the angle (rubeosis iridis).

Some of these cause transitory raised pressure and only require treatment while the condition is active, e.g. hyphema and iritis or continued corticosteroid use.

Damage to the trabecular meshwork caused by trauma means that intraocular pressure could rise many years after the initial injury. Thus all patients with significant eye trauma should have their intraocular pressure periodically checked by an optician.

Topical but not systemic steroid treatment can raise intraocular pressure in about 40 per cent of the population. It is important to be aware of this when prescribing steroid cream preparations to be used around the eye. Chronic usage should not occur unless intraocular pressure is being monitored and treated as necessary.

Pseudoexfoliation, where the capsule of the lens appears to be exfoliating, is quite common among Caucasians. It is actually amyloid material that coats the lens and clogs the trabecular meshwork, but the condition is not related to systemic amyloid disorders.

Treatment of secondary glaucomas is the same as that for open angle glaucoma.

Treatment of glaucoma

Treatment is focused on lowering intraocular pressure, and medical treatment with drops is the mainstay of treatment.

Drug	Main side effect
Beta-blockers (e.g. Timoptol 0.5%)	Exacerbation of COAD
Latanoprost	Conjunctival irritation
Dorzolomide	Conjunctivitis
Brimonidine	Ocular irritation
Pilocarpine	Pupil constriction

Beta-blockers such as Timoptol 0.5% twice daily are a common first-line drug, and are effective in lowering intraocular pressure. There are, however, several other drops that are used either singly or in conjunction with each other (see table). If intraocular pressure is not controlled by medical therapy, or if the disease progresses despite reasonable pressure control, most ophthalmologists would consider surgery.

Trabeculectomy

The purpose of this operation is to form a permanent fistula between the anterior chamber of the eye and the conjunctiva. This allows aqueous to leak out under the conjunctiva, thus lowering the intraocular pressure (Figure 20.6). Surgery is successful in 80–90 per cent of cases but will fail in some patients because of an excessive fibrotic healing response, which blocks up the fistula. In cases with a high risk of failure, antimetabolites (5-fluorouracil or mitomicin) are used intraoperatively to prevent fibrosis.

Patients are often operated on under local anaesthesia as day cases.

Figure 20.6 A bleb forms in the conjunctiva at the operating site where aqueous pools after escaping from the eye.

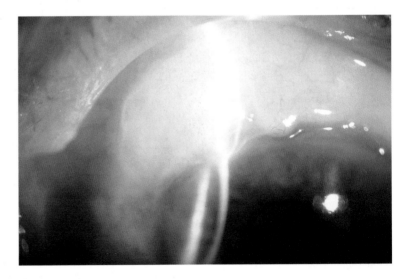

Postoperative treatment: Corticosteroid drops and dilating drops are routinely used for 2–4 months.

Complications: Complications surrounding over- or under-drainage of the fistula are common.

PIGMENTED RETINAL LESIONS

Fundal inspection forms part of an optician's general eye examination. Occasionally this will turn up an unexpected finding, commonly a pigmented lesion in the fundus. The unspoken concern is whether this represents early malignant melanoma.

Retinal naevi

About 1–2 per cent of the population have choroidal naevi. They are probably present at birth, and may grow during puberty. After this they should remain static in size. The potential for malignant transformation is extremely low, and so typical cases are usually discharged from further follow-up (Figure 20.7). More suspicious cases may be photographed and observed periodically. Any sign of growth changes the diagnosis to malignant melanoma.

Action

Non-urgent referral is indicated.

Figure 20.7 Typical cases are flat and covered with yellow/white drusen. Reproduced with permission from *Clinical Ophthalmology* by J. Kanski, 1999.

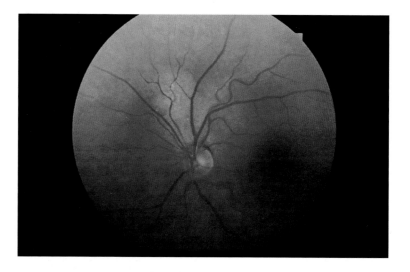

Malignant melanoma

Action

Urgent referral is indicated.

Presentation is usually during the sixth decade of life, either by chance as above or due to symptoms of a retinal detachment (Figure 20.8).

Treatment

Small tumours are treated with a plaque emitting radiation sutured to the sclera overlying the tumour. Larger tumours are treated by removal of the eye.

Figure 20.8 Melanoma causing a solid retinal detachment.
Reproduced with permission from *Clinical Ophthalmology* by J. Kanski, 1999.

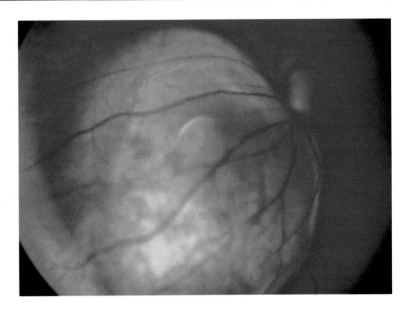

BLURRED VISION

The commonest causes are cataract and macular degeneration; however, three other rarer causes of blurred vision are worth mentioning here, as they are most likely to present from this source:

- Fuchs endothelial dystrophy
- Keratoconus
- Corneal dystrophies.

Fuchs endothelial dystrophy

This is an occasional finding in elderly patients with blurred vision. Commonly, there is also some associated nuclear sclerotic cataract. The corneal endothelium is a monolayer of cells that pump water from the cornea in order to maintain its clarity. Premature loss of significant numbers of these cells leads to corneal oedema and blurred vision.

> *Action*
>
> Cataract surgery may be indicated, but this will further reduce the endothelial cell population and make corneal oedema worse. Replacement endothelial cells can only be obtained by performing a corneal graft.

Keratoconus

Keratoconus is relatively rare, and is due to abnormal collagen in the cornea causing central thinning. Intraocular pressure then pushes the central cornea forward into a cone shape (Figure 20.9).

Figure 20.9 Keratoconus becomes evident during the second and third decades, and is associated with atopy and Down's syndrome. The shape of the cornea causes irregular astigmatism, blurring the patient's vision.

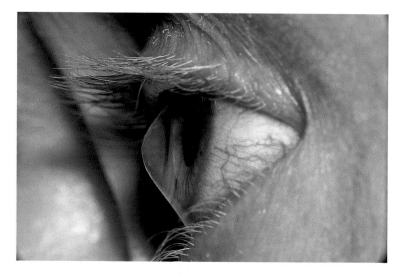

Action

In the early stages the optician will manage the condition with contact lenses, but in some cases the condition worsens to the extent that a corneal graft is required to restore normal corneal shape.

Corneal dystrophies

Corneal dystrophies are very rare and are caused by biochemical abnormalities leading to deposition of material in the cornea, which interrupts the patient's vision (Figure 20.10).

Action

Referral is indicated to decide on the appropriateness of corneal grafting.

Figure 20.10 Granular dystrophy. Other types include lattice dystrophy and macular dystrophy. Reproduced with permission from *Clinical Ophthalmology* by J. Kanski, 1999.

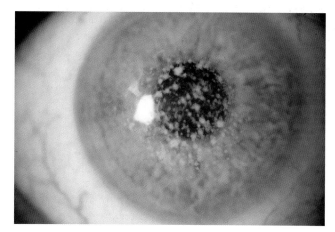

Figure 20.11 (a) A disc of clear cornea is cut from a donor. (b) A similarly-sized disc of diseased cornea is removed from the recipient eye. (c) The donor graft is then sutured in. Reproduced with permission from *Clinical Ophthalmology* by J. Kanski, 1999.

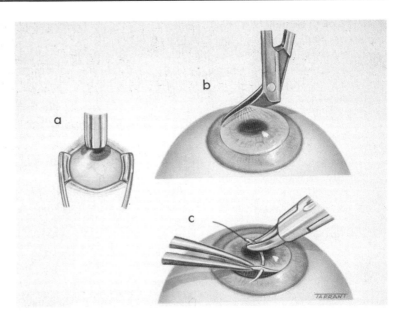

Corneal grafting (keratoplasty)

Corneal grafting involves replacing a diseased cornea with a healthy one from a deceased donor (Figure 20.11). Tissue matching is rarely required.

Postoperative treatment: Steroid drops are used postoperatively to reduce inflammation and prevent rejection. Drops may continue for a year or more.

Complications: Rejection still occurs in around 20 per cent of cases, and presents with uveitis (painful red eye) or blurred vision. These cases require urgent referral, as prompt treatment with corticosteroids can rescue the situation.

Part VII

General medicine

The eye and general medicine

This is a large topic, but fortunately most link-ups are rather obscure. Some of the less rare disorders are discussed in Chapter 30. The more common general medical diseases that affect the eye are:

- Diabetes (see Chapter 22)
- Rheumatoid arthritis
- Thyroid disease
- Multiple sclerosis
- Hypertension.

The eye's unique function allows the doctor to look into it through the corneal window and view living tissue. Functioning arteries and veins can be observed, as well as the effects of disease upon them. The eye is particularly susceptible to:

- Autoimmune diseases, including vasculitic conditions
- Diseases that affect the blood or blood vessels
- Diseases that affect the brain and brainstem.

Rheumatoid arthritis

The effects on the eye vary from mild to very severe. Many patients suffer from Sjögren's syndrome, which gives them a dry eye and mouth. The dry eye is irritating, and should be treated with artificial tears that should be instilled as often as required. If the dryness is severe, punctal occlusion should be considered.

> **Action**
>
> Patients whose symptoms cannot be controlled with simple eye lubrication should be referred.

For no known reason corneal thinning can suddenly occur which, despite treatment, melts the cornea, with eventual perforation of the eye. These cases are very frustrating to treat, and may require gluing of the corneal hole or even emergency corneal grafting to maintain the integrity of the eye.

Thyroid eye disease

Thyroid eye disease is most associated with hyperthyroidism and Graves' disease, but it can rarely occur in hypothyroid and even euthyroid states. Treatment of the thyroid status does not influence the eye disease. Thyroid eye disease can cause:

- Lid retraction
- Proptosis
- Double vision
- Optic neuropathy.

Multiple sclerosis

Some patients presenting with optic neuritis for the first time will go on to full-blown multiple sclerosis. Seventy per cent of known sufferers of multiple sclerosis show evidence of previous attacks of optic neuritis.

Hypertension

In general medical textbooks much is made of changes in the retina, such as silver and copper wiring. However, these changes are indistinguishable from normal ageing changes, and anyway the author has always found that diagnosing and monitoring hypertension is easier with a sphygmomanometer rather than an ophthalmoscope!

Having said that, malignant hypertension is sometimes diagnosed via the ophthalmoscope. Patients with blood pressures typically around 230/140 often complain of headache and slightly blurred vision. Because headache is such a non-specific symptom, the focus for diagnosis may fall on the eyes. The fundal picture is dramatic, with cotton-wool spots, disc oedema, tiny thin arteries, and bulging veins (Figure 21.1). Patients with long-standing hypertension associated with renal disease often display a more exudative picture, with scattered, hard exudates.

> **Action**
>
> Patients with malignant hypertension are in danger of a vascular catastrophe, and require urgent control of blood pressure.

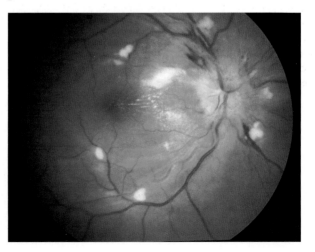

Figure 21.1 Malignant hypertension. Reproduced with permission from *Clinical Ophthalmology* by J. Kanski, 1999.

Diabetic retinopathy

In the United Kingdom there are approximately 1 million diabetics, of whom 20 per cent are insulin dependent and 80 per cent non-insulin dependent. Blindness amongst diabetics is 10 times the rate amongst the general public, and diabetic retinopathy is the most common reason for blindness in the working age group.

NATURAL HISTORY

Diabetes wreaks its damage on the body through its effects on both large vessels (increased myocardial infarction and stroke) and small vessels (nephropathy, neuropathy, retinopathy). In the eye, initial damage is to the small vessel wall and results in microaneurysms with subsequent leakage of blood, lipoprotein and fluid ('background diabetic retinopathy'; Figure 22.1). Clinically, this is observed as:

- Scattered haemorrhages
- Hard exudates
- Retinal oedema.

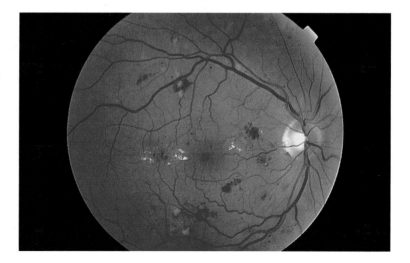

Figure 22.1 Background diabetic retinopathy. Scattered haemorrhages and hard exudates are evident. Retinal oedema requires binocular indirect ophthalmoscopy to be appreciated.

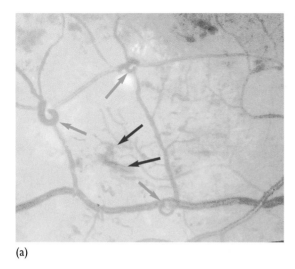

(a)

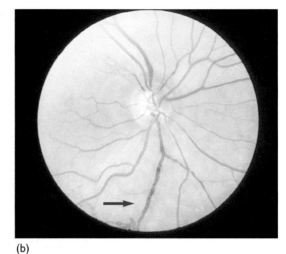

(b)

Figure 22.2 Preproliferative retinopathy. (a) Venous looping (green arrows) and intraretinal microvascular abnormalities (blue arrows). The microvascular abnormalities are vascular shunts, which appear as wispy, thin vessels connecting larger vessels. (b) Venous beading (blue arrow).

If this affects the macular area, associated swelling in the retina reduces visual acuity ('maculopathy'). Background diabetic retinopathy is commonly present at diagnosis of maturity-onset diabetes, but in juvenile-onset diabetes only 50 per cent of patients will have retinopathy after 10 years, while 90 per cent will be affected after 20 years.

As blood vessel damage progresses capillary closure occurs, inducing ischaemia by preventing the supply of oxygen to that area of retina. With increasing ischaemia, further retinal changes develop (Figure 22.2):

- Cotton wool spots (microinfarcts)
- Large blot haemorrhages
- Venous beading and venous loops
- Intraretinal vascular abnormalities.

Figure 22.3 New vessels growing on the disc. Reproduced with permission from *Clinical Ophthalmology* by J. Kanski, 1999.

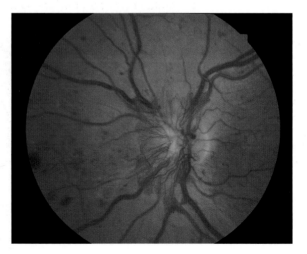

Figure 22.4 New vessels growing elsewhere on the retina.

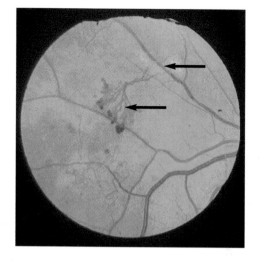

This appearance is referred to as 'preproliferative retinopathy'.
  Once approximately one-quarter of the retina is ischaemic, further changes occur:

- New vessels grow at the disc (Figure 22.3)
- New vessels grow on the retina (Figure 22.4)
- Fibrotic membranes develop along with new vessel growth
- New vessels develop on the iris.

This appearance is referred to as 'proliferative retinopathy'.

Complications: There are several reasons why vision can be lost in diabetic eye disease:

- Severe macular oedema from long-standing maculopathy
- Ischaemic retina at the macula (Figure 22.5)

Figure 22.5 Fluorescein angiogram of ischaemic diabetic maculopathy. The dark holes in the angiogram represent areas of no blood perfusion and ischaemia. The frost-like appearance on the blood vessels represents capillary closure. Reproduced with permission from *Clinical Ophthalmology* by J. Kanski, 1999.

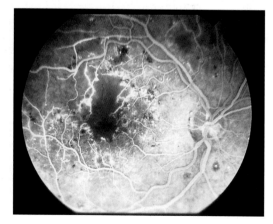

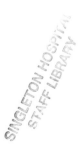

- Vitreous haemorrhage from ruptured new vessels (Figure 22.6) – this will normally clear spontaneously over the next 3–4 months
- Fibrotic membranes associated with new vessel formation causing tractional retinal detachment (Figure 22.7)
- Intractable glaucoma associated with new vessel growth on the iris (Figure 22.8).

Figure 22.6 Diagram showing haemorrhage caused by traction on the new vessels.

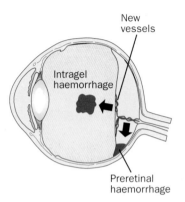

Figure 22.7 Fibrotic membranes over the optic disc. Note the lines of traction across the macula. Reproduced with permission from *Clinical Ophthalmology* by J. Kanski, 1999.

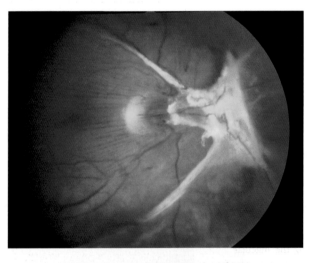

Figure 22.8 Rubeosis iridis. The new blood vessels on the iris block the trabecular meshwork, causing glaucoma.

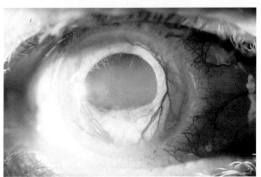

CARE OF THE DIABETIC PATIENT

Action

Any signs of maculopathy or ischaemia of the retina should be referred to the local eye department for evaluation and possible treatment.

Rigorous control of blood glucose levels is the best way of delaying disease progression. The importance of this issue should not distract attention from control of any hypertension, anaemia or poor renal function. All patients should be encouraged to refrain from smoking. Examinations of the retina should occur every 9 months to a year. This can be done either at the optician, by fundal photography at the local diabetic department, or indeed by the general practitioner.

TREATMENT OF RETINOPATHY

The mainstay of treatment is argon laser photocoagulation. This is delivered via a slit lamp as a day case procedure. Some patients find the procedure painful and have difficulty in holding their eyelids open against the intense flash of laser light. In these rare cases, a local anaesthetic injection can be given beforehand.

Pan-retinal photocoagulation destroys some of the visual field, and patients should be warned that treatment might result in failure to maintain the standard demanded to hold a driving licence (see Chapter 28).

Maculopathy

Maculopathy is treated with light argon laser treatment. The laser beam can either be aimed at a leaking point in the retina, or for more generalized oedema a scattered grid pattern across

Figure 22.9 Appearance following pan-retinal photocoagulation. Round white laser scars can be seen surrounding the macular area. Reproduced with permission from *Clinical Ophthalmology* by J. Kanski, 1999.

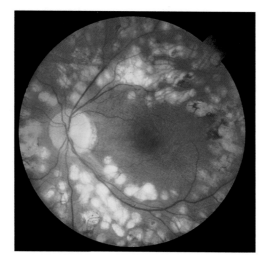

the macula is employed. The former is usually very successful, while the latter is generally less so.

Ischaemia

The characteristic fundal changes can be quantified by fluorescein angiography (Figure 22.5). The argon laser is again the mainstay of treatment, but it is used in a destructive capacity. The burns are meant to kill the underlying retina and therefore reduce the ischaemic load. Treatment involves scattering 2000–4000 laser burns around the peripheral retina ('pan-retinal photocoagulation') while sparing the macular area (Figure 22.9). In most cases, new vessel growth can be reversed with involution of the vessels.

Vitreous haemorrhage

Persistent haemorrhage that does not clear can be removed by vitrectomy. An endolaser can be used during the operation to apply further pan-retinal photocoagulation.

Traction detachment and opaque membranes

The fibrotic membranes can be segmented and traction relieved using special scissors after vitrectomy has been carried out (Figure 22.10).

Figure 22.10 Principles of vitrectomy for traction detachment. (a) Fibrous bands are cut. (b) Pan-retinal photocoagulation using an internal laser. Reproduced with permission from *Clinical Ophthalmology* by J. Kanski, 1999.

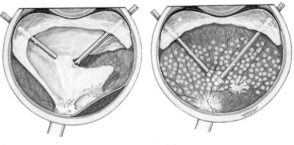

(a)   (b)

Part VIII

Childhood eye conditions

Introduction to childhood eye conditions

Sometimes the most obvious clinical feature of a patient's complaint is his or her age. Many eye disorders are unique to children, and for these reasons they are grouped in a section of their own. The disorders are grouped, as in the rest of the book, by the presenting complaint:

- Change in appearance of the face
    Acutely inflamed (orbital cellulitis)
    Uninflamed (lumps and bumps, prominent eyes, ptosis
- Change in appearance of the eye
    Acutely inflamed (acute swelling of conjunctiva)
    Uninflamed (squint, white pupil reflex, abnormal eye movements, increased size)
- Reduced vision and the blind child
- Watering/red/sticky eyes.

In young children the visual system is still immature, and to understand some of the effects of poor vision or squint some understanding of visual development is required.

VISUAL DEVELOPMENT IN CHILDREN

Most predators, including humans, have evolved faces with both eyes pointing forward, while those preyed upon have evolved eyes on the sides of the head to give themselves a panoramic view and early warning of impending danger. The predators have evolved their facial anatomy with one purpose in mind – three-dimensional vision (stereopsis). Two eyes locked onto an object from slightly different positions (exactly the same arrangement as a weapons guidance system locking onto a target from two coordinates) allow depth perception, a vital advantage in catching prey.

A baby can't walk, talk or kick a football. These skills are acquired over a number of years as the child's neurological system matures. The same is true of the visual system, with full maturity only occurring around 7 years of age. At birth, an inborn reflex normally brings the image of an object onto both foveae. Over time, continual practice of this reflex is cemented into the ability to perceive depth (stereopsis). This system can break down in two situations:

- If one eye has poor vision
    Congenital cataract
    High refractive error
    Ptosis covering the visual axis
    Other occult pathology, e.g. retinoblastoma
- If one eye is squinting.

In the former case, the brain ignores the image from the poor eye and concentrates on the good eye. The abandoned eye then develops a convergent squint (eye turning in). In the latter case, logic would dictate that if each eye were pointing in a different direction the brain would receive two different images from each fovea and therefore experience double vision. To prevent this, young children with immature visual systems have the ability to suppress the image from the squinting eye (this ability is lost after the age of 7, and new cases of squinting later than this age do result in double vision). Suppression to prevent double vision is only needed when both eyes are open, and so the visual acuity of the squinting eye if tested on its own is actually normal. If, however, suppression continues for a few weeks or more, the visual acuity in the squinting eye when tested on its own starts to deteriorate (amblyopia). If left untreated, vision in the squinting eye is likely to fall as low as 6/60 or worse. It goes without saying that in both cases stereopsis does not develop.

AMBLYOPIA

This is a state of reduced visual acuity in one eye that results from chronic suppression of the visual image of this eye by the brain. This reduction in acuity secondary to suppression only occurs in the first few years of life, and does not occur once the visual system has reached maturity at around the age of 7 years. Similarly, amblyopia is only treatable while the visual system remains immature i.e. before the age of 7 years.

Treatment

Initial assessment of squints and treatment of amblyopia is carried out by orthoptists, who are visual development and muscle balance specialists based at the eye department. The visual decline in the poor or squinting eye can usually be halted if the child is less than 7 years old.

Figure 23.1 Patching. The child is prevented from using the good eye.

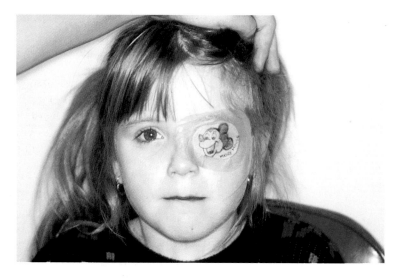

Once all impediments to good vision (e.g. cataract, ptosis) have been removed and any refractive errors corrected with glasses, the child should have patching treatment. This involves putting a patch on the good eye, thereby forcing the child to use the poor eye for vision (Figure 23.1). By this method the vision in the poor eye can be restored but, alas, even if the eyes are realigned by early surgery stereopsis does not usually develop. Instead, when both eyes are open, suppression of the poor eye continues but at least the vision remains good as a result of treatment for the amblyopia. These children require follow-up until they reach visual maturity to ensure that amblyopia does not reoccur. After visual maturity, amblyopia cannot develop. The treated eye therefore effectively becomes a spare eye, and the benefit of this is enjoyed should some disaster destroy the vision of the other good eye. The patient who had amblyopia treated as a child will enjoy good vision in the remaining eye, while the patient who had no treatment will have poor vision of 6/60 or worse.

Changes of the face

ACUTELY INFLAMED

Orbital cellulites

Orbital cellulitis is an infection of the soft tissues behind the orbital septum, and the resulting oedema restricts eye movements and causes a painful proptosis. Most cases occur in children and young adults and are frequently related to sinus disease (Figure 24.1).

Figure 24.1 Orbital cellulitis. The eye is shut, but if the lids are forced open eye movements will be very restricted.

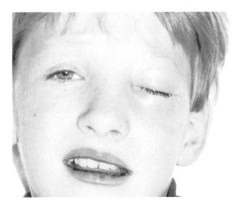

> *Action*
>
> Patients do not look well, and they need hospital admission for intra-venous antibiotics and evaluation for potential abscess drainage.

UNINFLAMED

Lumps and bumps

Capillary haemangiomas

Also known as strawberry naevi, capillary haemangiomas are relatively rare. They are hamartomas (overgrowths of normal tissue native to that location), but are worrying for parents as their appearance at birth or in the first few months of life is

Figure 24.2 Capillary haemangioma. The eyelid is a common site, and large tumours may cause amblyopia by obscuring the visual pathway of that eye.

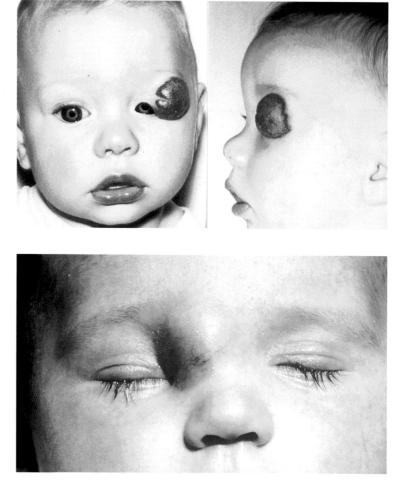

Figure 24.3 Buried capillary haemangioma.

followed by a period of rapid growth (Figure 24.2). Occasionally they may be buried below the skin, giving a bluish tinge to an evident mass (Figure 24.3).

Action

Capillary haemangiomas resolve spontaneously, but over some years. Intralesional injection with corticosteroids can accelerate resolution and may be necessary if amblyopia develops. If there is concern regarding normal visual development, then referral is indicated.

Dermoid cyst

Presentation is in infancy with a painless nodule most commonly located superotemporally (Figure 24.4). The cyst is

Figure 24.4 Dermoid cyst. Reproduced with permission from *Clinical Ophthalmology* by J. Kanski, 1999.

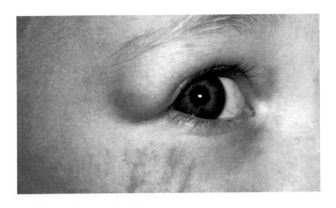

a choristoma (overgrowth of normal tissue foreign to that location), and is caused by embryological displacement of dermal tissue into a subcutaneous position.

> **Action**
>
> Referral for excision is indicated if cosmesis is poor. This is best done just before the child starts school..

Prominent eyes (proptosis)

This is rare, but is always a serious complaint in a child and requires urgent investigation. The differential diagnosis includes:

- Rhabdomyosarcoma – a rare malignant muscle tumour with peak incidence at the age of 7 years
- Orbital encephalocoele – the herniation of intracranial contents into the orbit via a bony defect in the orbital wall
- Retinoblastoma – a rare malignant retinal tumour with peak incidence at the age of 2 years
- Deep orbital capillary haemangioma.

Changes of the eye

INFLAMED

Acute swelling of the conjunctiva

This can be quite dramatic, and usually follows after the child has been playing in the grass outside. It is an acute allergic reaction, and is characterized by dramatic oedema of the conjunctiva but with a normal bright cornea (Figure 25.1).

Figure 25.1 Acute conjunctival swelling.

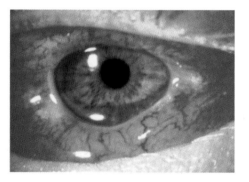

> *Action*
>
> No action is required apart from reassuring the parents, who are usually extremely anxious.

UNINFLAMED

Squint (strabismus)

There are several types of childhood squint:

- Paralytic, which is extremely rare and an easily excluded diagnosis with the observation of otherwise normal eye movements
- Non-paralytic, which is the common or garden squint

Convergent squint ('esotropia') – the eye turns in; this occurs in 80 per cent of cases and may be constant (present for near and distance) or accommodative (present only for near, and often only apparent when the child concentrates on a small picture held at reading distance)

Divergent squint ('exotropia') – the eye turns out; this occurs in 20 per cent of cases.

Why are squints important?

Squints are significant because of:

- Poor cosmesis
- Reduced vision in the squinting eye (amblyopia or 'lazy eye')
- Occult ocular pathology.

While cosmetic issues can be tackled at any time, the results of amblyopia treatment are best when treatment is started early. Ideally both issues should be tackled before the child goes to school, where name-calling either due to a manifest squint or the presence of a patch can be damaging. The squint itself can occasionally be caused by occult ocular pathology such as congenital cataract or retinoblastoma, and so all cases of squint seen in the hospital will have a thorough fundal examination.

Examination

Some squints are cosmetically obvious, but others are more subtle and are sometimes not noticed until amblyopia is discovered at a school eye test. Divergent squints are often difficult to detect because they tend to be intermittent, with the eyes appearing straight most of the time. They are often noticed by the parents from a distance – e.g. from across a room. Another clue is the tendency habitually to close one eye in sunlight.

Four tests in the primary care setting are particularly helpful in detecting squint:

- Corneal reflexes
- The cover test
- The accommodative target (useful in detecting accommodative squints)
- Eye movements.

Corneal reflexes: Shining a torch into the patient's eyes allows the corneal reflections to be observed. If the reflections are in

Figure 25.2 Convergent squint. Note the position of the corneal reflections (white dots on the cornea).

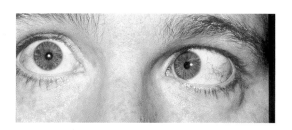

the same spot in both pupils a squint is not present. However, if the corneal reflection is not in the same place in both eyes a squint is clearly manifest (Figure 25.2).

The cover test: This test helps confirm what has been deduced from the corneal reflections. An object of interest is placed 30 cm from the child, and a cover is then put over the normal eye while the other eye is observed (Figure 25.3). If there is a squint then the eye swivels round to fixate on the object (Figure 25.4), but if there is no squint the eye does not move because it is already fixating on the object.

Figure 25.3 The cover test. An object is held in front of the child while one eye is covered.

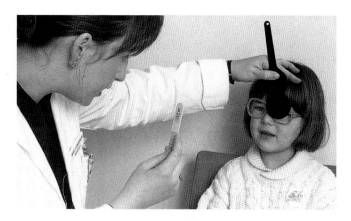

Figure 25.4 Confirmation of a convergent squint in the case show in Figure 25.1. A cover obscures the good eye, and the squinting eye has swivelled out to take up fixation on the object of interest.

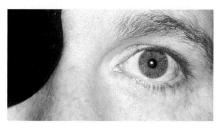

The accommodative target: This is useful for children of 2 years and upward, as the target must captivate their attention. A small picture 2–3 mm in size is used as a target, and this is placed in front of the patient at reading distance. A squint will become apparent if the child has an accommodative convergent squint.

Eye movements: Normal ocular motility excludes paralytic squint.

Presentation

Currently, children are screened several times during their early life. There are plans afoot, however, to substitute the last four checks with one examination performed by an orthoptist during the early school years.

Checks are made by:

- The GP
      6-week check
- The health visitor
      7-month check
      18-month check
      3+ preschool check, which includes a test of visual acuity (Sheridan Gardiner method – see Chapter 2)
- The school nurse
      School nurse (these are further checks of visual acuity)
        4–5-year-old check
        8-year-old check
        11-year-old check.

Most referrals are generated from these screening visits. At the 6-week check, constant squints will occasionally be present (they are large and obvious) and these should be referred. More commonly, however, the mother may report roving eye movements or intermittent squint. These cases usually resolve, and referral is only indicated if problems persist at the 7-month check.

Occasionally worried mothers will bring their child to the surgery between the 18-month and 3+ screening visits. If parents report a squint at this age, especially if it is related to looking at picture books, ignore their concern at your peril. They are usually right.

Treatment

The aims of treatment in the hospital are:

- To exclude other pathology such as cataract or retinoblastoma

- To treat amblyopia and any refractive errors
- To improve cosmesis.

If a squint is cosmetically upsetting, surgery may be required to straighten the eyes. This is best done before the child goes to school and nicknames are acquired.

Squint surgery is like pitching a tent. In this scenario, lengthening and shortening of the guy ropes manipulates the amount by which the tent lists. In the same way, altering the length of the extraocular muscles manipulates the position of the eye. Surgery is usually a day case procedure, despite involving general anaesthesia. A certain amount of experience and guesswork is required to estimate the correct amount of manipulation, and it is not uncommon for a second operation to needed for the perfect result.

Pseudosquint

This is caused by an optical illusion attributable to a broad epicanthic fold. The illusion is enhanced if the child looks slightly to one side (Figure 25.5), and this is often what the mothers report – an intermittent squint apparent when the child looks out of the corner of the eye. The suspicion that the eye is normal can be confirmed by symmetrical corneal reflections and a normal cover test.

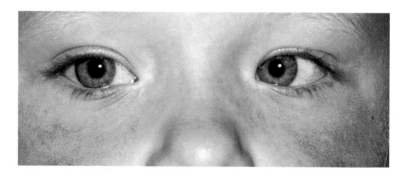

Figure 25.5 Pseudosquint. The left eye appears to be turning in, but in fact the child is looking to the right. Note the symmetry of the corneal reflexes.

White pupil reflex (leukocoria)

Action

Immediate referral is necessary.

Leukocoria is a rare but important presentation (Figure 25.6). It is the commonest mode of presentation of retinoblastoma, which is a rare, malignant tumour of the retina that is life threatening but eminently treatable. Around 20 per cent of patients will present with a convergent squint.

Figure 25.6 Leukocoria caused by retinoblastoma.

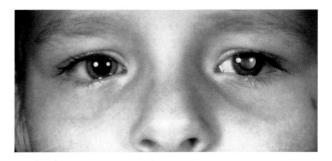

Unusual eye movements

Action
Nystagmus is always an important sign that requires urgent investigation.

Occasionally children will be brought in with nystagmus, which is a repetitive to-and-fro involuntary movement of the eyes. It commonly occurs in children with bilaterally poor vision.

Size of the eye

Action
Immediate referral is necessary.

Enlargement of the eyes is another rare but important presentation. Parents do not usually notice if both eyes are enlarged, but if only one is enlarged it is more obvious. Congenital glaucoma is the most likely diagnosis, with high intraocular pressure expanding the scleral shell.

Reduced vision and the blind child

REDUCED VISUAL ACUITY

Action

Referral to the eye department is indicated for treatment of any refractive error or amblyopia.

This is commonly discovered at the screening visits performed by the health visitor or school nurse. A squint should be searched for, utilizing corneal reflections, cover testing and accommodative target. The causes of decreased vision are usually:

- Amblyopia secondary to a squint
- Refractive error
- Rarely, occult pathology.

BLINDNESS

Action

Referral is indicated to establish the cause, some of which (e.g. congenital cataract) are treatable.

Some unfortunate children will have been born with conditions causing poor vision. The mother often becomes worried in the first few months of life, as the child shows no apparent interest in fixating on anything but instead demonstrates continually wandering eyes. Eventually such children will develop nystagmus.

Functional blindness

Action

Referral is indicated, as just occasionally a genuine case emerges. For the majority of patients, though, good vision is usually coaxed out of them at the clinic visit and eye examination, including pupil reactions, is normal. They are usually discharged after one visit with no further investigation.

This is very common in the 9–14 years age group, especially amongst girls. The story varies from bilateral complete blindness to central scotomas and unilateral tunnel vision. The most striking feature is the relaxed attitude of the patient and the wound-up nature of the mother (presumably the main point of the exercise).

Watering/sticky/red eyes

WATERING EYES IN A BABY

Watering and sticky eyes are common amongst young babies, and are caused by failure of the nasolacrimal duct to canalize. Parents describe having to remove mucus from the eyes several times a day. Examination shows matter on the eyelids, but the conjunctiva is not normally inflamed.

Action

Spontaneous canalization is the norm, but if symptoms persist over 15 months then referral for probing of the nasolacrimal duct is indicated. In the meantime, parents should be instructed to remove mucopus from the eyes periodically. Topical chloramphenicol is of limited value, but may be useful if there is overt infection of the mucoid material.

Congenital glaucoma

Watering associated with photophobia and eye rubbing is suggestive of congenital glaucoma. This is very rare, but requires urgent attention. Occasionally the eyes are enlarged, but clouding of the cornea is the most frequent sign recognized by the parents (Figure 27.1).

Figure 27.1 Congenital glaucoma. High intraocular pressure causes enlargement of the eyes, known as bupthalmos ('ox eye'), and corneal clouding.

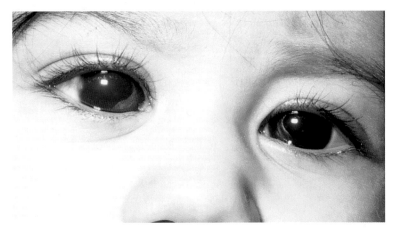

RED EYES

Most cases of red eyes in children are due to conjunctivitis. Dendritic ulceration and corneal ulcers are extremely rare, but become more common in the later teenage years.

Vernal keratoconjunctivitis

<table>
<tr><td>

Action

Referral to the eye department is indicated, as long-term corticosteroid treatment is usually necessary. The disease usually burns itself out in early adulthood.

</td></tr>
</table>

Vernal keratoconjunctivitis (spring catarrh) is an uncommon disorder related to atopy that causes very uncomfortable, red, intensely itchy, photophobic and watery eyes in children between the ages of 5 and 18 years. Presentation during the hay fever season is typical although not universal. Eversion of the upper lid reveals giant papillae, which appear like cobblestones on the conjunctiva (Figure 26.2). These may abrade the cornea, causing a central 'shield ulcer' to develop.

Figure 27.2 Vernal keratoconjunctivitis. Giant cobblestone papillae are seen on everting the upper lid.

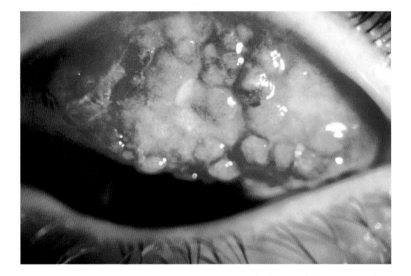

Part IX

Miscellany

Visual standards

VISUAL IMPAIRMENT REGISTRATION

Only one in three patients who are eligible for registration are actually registered. Registration triggers vital support from social services and voluntary groups, which may take the form of:

- Practical help and emotional support
    Home care and adaptations to the home
    Tape and large-print library facilities
    Visual aids
    Social worker visits
    Help in learning to get about safely
- Financial benefits
- Tax allowances
- Disability living allowance or attendance allowance
- Housing benefit
- Free NHS prescriptions and sight tests
- Railcard concessions
- Telephone concessions.

Blind registration

To be registered blind:

- Vision must be worse than 3/60 in both eyes, *or*
- Vision must be worse than 6/60 in both eyes with a restricted visual field.

Partially sighted registration

There is no formal statute defining partially sighted registration, but guidelines suggest:

- Vision worse than 6/60 in both eyes, *or*
- Vision worse than 6/18 in both eyes with a restricted visual field, *or*

● Hemianopias and quadrantinopias of both eyes regardless of visual acuity.

Note that people with only one normally functioning eye are not eligible for partially sighted registration, a fact that some patients find difficult to understand.

VISUAL STANDARD REQUIRED FOR DRIVING

An individual's fitness to drive is determined by the Driver and Vehicle Licensing Authority (DVLA). A leaflet (form D100), available from the post office, explains the standards required for various licences. Licence holders are obliged to inform the DVLA (and their motor insurers) if they develop a medical condition or experience worsening of an existing condition that might affect their fitness to drive. In this instance the DVLA may ask an optician to provide the relevant visual data to allow a decision to be made regarding whether or not to continue an individual's licence.

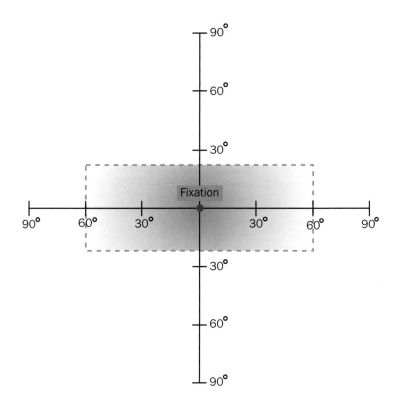

Figure 28.1 The area of clear visual field required to obtain a driving licence.

Criteria for a private licence

- Central acuity – with corrected acuity a person must be capable of reading a car registration number at a distance of 20.5 m (this equates to approximately 6/12 vision)
- Visual field (this is tested with both eyes open) – the rectangle of visual field shown (Figure 28.1) should have no significant field defects. Patients with hemianopia or quadrantinopia do not meet this visual standard.
- Double vision – if a person has double vision, one eye must be patched to achieve single vision and a suitable adaptation period should be allowed.

Possession of only one functioning eye is not a bar to holding a private licence, but it is a bar to new applications for a public service or heavy goods licence. Again an adaptation period of perhaps 3 months is suggested for patients who have experienced recent visual loss in one eye.

Sample cases

QUESTIONS

1. The optician's letter states:
   'this man has a cataract in the left eye and I have advised him to seek a specialist opinion'.
   His visual acuity is 6/9 right and 6/12 left.
   What do you do as a GP?
   Are there any options?

2. Ten weeks after uncomplicated cataract surgery, a patient requests a further prescription of G maxidex. He missed his postoperative review.
   What are you going to do?

3. One year after cataract surgery, a patient complains of gradual deterioration in vision in the operated eye.
   What is the likely cause?
   What do you do?

4. A 50-year-old man notices a single black object in the field of vision of his left eye. It moves on eye movements.
   What is the likely cause?
   What will you do?
   What features would cause concern?

5. A 28-year-old female presents with a smooth, round swelling in the left upper lid. It has been present for 2 months.
   What is the likely diagnosis?
   What do you do?

6. A 20-year-old woman presents with bilateral red eyes that are gritty and burning. Discharge is evident on the lashes.
   What is the likely diagnosis?
   What else could it be?

7. A 24-year-old man presents with a painful red left eye that has been present for 5 days and has been getting worse every day. He is quite photophobic.

What do you do?
What conditions would you consider?

8. An 80-year-old woman complains of a very painful eye along with a feeling of nausea of 2 days' duration. On examination the eye is red.
What condition do you want to exclude?
How do you do this?

9. A 75-year-old man complains of sudden loss of vision in one eye. Visual acuity is 'hand movements' only.
What are the likely causes?
What condition do you want to exclude?
How do you do this?

ANSWERS

1. It seems reasonable to assume that the patient has cataract and that routine referral to the eye department for consideration of cataract surgery is indicated. However, other issues are important and worth consideration. Chief amongst these is whether the patient actually feels a need for cataract surgery. Referral is not always necessary. Lifestyle issues such as the ability to drive, perform a job or care for a relative may have special importance and deserve mention in the letter to the eye department. You may feel that some cases deserve priority status. Extreme old age and poor health are not necessarily bars to having cataract surgery.

2. Maxidex is a corticosteroid drop commonly used after cataract surgery to control postoperative inflammation. Under normal circumstances it is only used four times a day for about 2–3 weeks, and it is generally stopped at the postoperative visit. Therefore the request should be denied, especially if the eye is white and uninflamed in an asymptomatic patient. Early review in the hospital should be arranged.

3. About 20–30 per cent of patients will develop posterior capsule opacification following cataract surgery. Blistering of the posterior capsule caused by proliferation of residual lens fibres will cause gradual blurring of the vision. The other common possibility is macular degeneration, which is also likely in this age group. The diagnosis can be confirmed by examining the red reflex, which is abnormal in posterior capsule opacification. Patients should be referred for laser treatment, which can open up the capsule and restore normal vision (see Figures 7.7, 7.8).

4. Posterior vitreous detachment is a common condition, and patients describe symptoms of floaters. These can be multiple or single. Single floaters are often described as a cobweb or a fly that patients wish they could wipe from their field of vision. Patients should be referred according to the guidelines outlined in Chapter 9. Worrying features suggestive of associated retinal detachment are decreased visual acuity and a history of a 'storm' of floaters. These cases require urgent referral to an eye casualty department.

5. The most likely diagnosis is that of a meibomium cyst or chalazion. These will often involute of their own accord, but referral for incision and drainage is warranted in persistent cases.

6. Bacterial conjunctivitis is the most likely diagnosis, and should be treated with chloramphenicol drops used every 2 hours and supplemented with chloramphenicol ointment at night. The critical feature of the case is the presence of pus, which excludes many of the serious causes of a red eye. Examination of the cornea will exclude a corneal ulcer, which may be a possibility if the patient is a contact lens wearer. Other possible diagnoses to entertain are viral conjunctivitis with secondary bacterial infection, and the possibility of chlamydial infection in the sexually active.

7. The absence of pus and the increasing pain are worrying signs. The visual acuity may well be affected as well. Using Figure 16.1a, the most likely diagnoses are acute glaucoma, dendritic ulcer, iritis or scleritis. Acute glaucoma can be excluded because the patient is too young, and scleritis is very rare. This leaves dendritic ulcer and iritis as the main contenders. Dendritic ulcer can be diagnosed by staining the cornea with fluorescein dye. Urgent referral to the eye casualty department is indicated.

8. This patient has a red and very painful eye, and the first thought should be to exclude acute glaucoma. Examining the pupil can achieve this. In acute glaucoma, the pupil is mid-dilated and unreactive to light. Digital palpation of the eye will reveal a stony hardness.

9. Given the patient's age, vascular causes are top of the list. These would include:

    * Central retinal vein occlusion
    * Central retinal artery occlusion
    * Anterior ischaemic optic neuropathy
    * Macular haemorrhage
    * Vitreous haemorrhage.

Examination of the visual field along with examination of the retina (through a dilated pupil) will narrow the diagnosis (see Figure 5.1). If retinal artery occlusion or ischaemic optic neuropathy are suspected, underlying giant cell arteritis must be excluded. This is best done by direct enquiry, looking for the classic symptoms of:

- Malaise and weight loss
- Scalp tenderness
- Pain on chewing or talking.

Glossary of words, drugs and rarities

Aniridia: Congenital absence of the iris, usually associated with glaucoma.

Anisocoria: Different sized pupils.

Anisometropia: Difference in refraction between the two eyes.

Ankylosing spondylitis: An autoimmune condition of gradual fusing of the thoracic spine; many patients will also suffer from acute iritis.

Asteroid hyalitis: Intergalactic-like bodies suspended in the vitreous. They have a dramatic appearance and, astonishingly, are asymptomatic (Figure 30.1).

Figure 30.1 Asteroid hyalitis. An incidental finding on ophthalmoscopy.

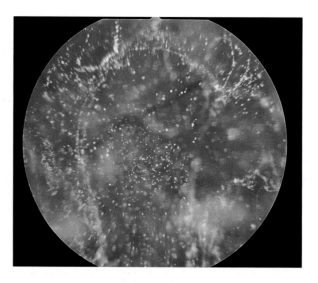

Chloroquine retinopathy: Chloroquine is used for the treatment of certain collagen disorders, and for prophylaxis against malaria. High dosage can cause a retinopathy, which affects the visual acuity, and so hydroxychloroquine (which is less toxic) is usually preferred.

CHRPE: Acronym for congenital hypertrophy of the retinal pigment epithelium. This is densely pigmented retinal spots that are often confused with retinal naevi. Occasionally they appear in clumps and look like animal tracks (hence the alternative titles of 'bear track' and 'cat's paw' pigmentation). It does not require further follow-up.

Coloboma: Congenital defect that can cause complete gaps of the uveal tract in the inferior quadrant (Figure 30.2).

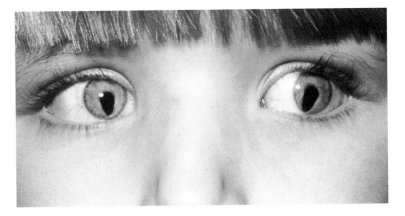

Figure 30.2 Coloboma of the iris, giving a keyhole appearance.

Cytomegalovirus retinitis: The result of cytomegalovirus infection of the retina. This only occurs in extreme immunocompromised states, and is particularly associated with end-stage AIDS (Figure 30.3).

Enucleation: Removal of the whole eye.

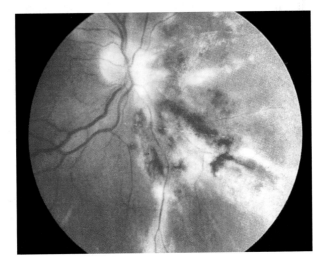

Figure 30.3 CMV retinitis, sometimes described as having a 'pizza pie' appearance.

Epiphora: Latinized name for watering of the eye.

Evisceration: Removal of the eye contents, leaving behind the scleral shell.

Exenteration: Removal of the contents of the orbit right down to the bone. The defect is usually lined with skin. This technique is used for advanced malignancy.

Guttae: Latin plural of 'gutta', meaning drop. It precedes the name of a drug prescribed in drop form (e.g. guttae (G.) chloramphenicol).

Internuclear ophthalmoplegia: Abnormal horizontal eye movements occurring in both eyes, with nystagmus affecting the eyes in lateral gaze. Disruption of communications between the right and left eye in the brainstem is the cause. In young patients this is due to demyelination (usually multiple sclerosis), and in the elderly to a brainstem stroke.

Leukaemia: This can produce iris changes as well as haemorrhages in the retina.

Macroaneurysm: Dilatation of the retinal arteries caused by hypertension. Leakage and oedema can affect the macula. If so, an argon laser can destroy the aneurysm.

Myotonic dystrophy: Autosomal dominant condition with muscle wasting of the face leading to a mournful expression. Patients also have ptosis and presenile cataract formation.

Oculentum: Latin for 'ointment'. This precedes the name of a drug in ointment form (e.g. Oculentum (Oc.) chloramphenicol).

Optic disc drusen: Autosomal dominant condition where hyaline material is superficially buried in the substance of the disc. Drusen can give the appearance of papilloedema and may also cause visual field defects; otherwise they are benign and require no treatment.

Retinitis pigmentosa: Inherited condition that causes night blindness and a constricted field of vision. The onset is variable, but commonly starts during the second decade.

Retinopathy of prematurity: A complication of low birthweight premature babies. Retinal development is abnormal, with potential blinding consequences. Early intervention with laser treatment may prevent retinal detachment and blindness.

Scotoma: A depression in the retinal sensitivity discovered on visual field testing. Absolute scotomas are areas of no sensitivity (e.g. the optic disc).

Still's disease: A rare disorder of childhood causing arthritis. Some children also suffer from an asymptomatic uveitis.

Tobacco–alcohol amblyopia: Heavy consumers of both substances who forget to eat as well can suffer from loss of central acuity. Parenteral hydroxycobalamine can halt the macular decline.

Toxoplasmosis: This can be picked up during pregnancy – usually from eating undercooked meat rather than from cats, as is popularly thought. Infection during the first trimester will lead to spontaneous abortion; infection during the second trimester usually results in mental retardation; and infection during the third trimester leads to bouts of posterior uveitis in the offspring. The infection has little effect on adults unless they are immunocompromised.

Index